Emotional Intelligence in Dentistry

This book is a comprehensive guide for dental professionals (from undergraduates to experienced practitioners) to understand and apply the core skills of Emotional Intelligence to enhance their personal and professional success. EQ relates to how an individual can understand and manage their own emotional needs as well as recognise and deal with the needs of others and the skills to do this. For dental professionals, these are important skills to have, as every interaction with a patient requires the ability to connect with them emotionally in a positive way. Research shows us that those who can put their EQ skills into practice are more successful and happier in life.

The book is pragmatic in nature, drawing on real-life case studies from dentists in the field. This book looks at the application of the most up-to-date research on EQ that will make a direct impact on the practice of dentistry.

T0291115

Emotional Intelligence in Dentistry

"Open Wide" – The Five Critical Skills to Take Dentists from Good to Great

Edited by
Mary Collins
CPsychol, EdD, MSc, BA, EMCC

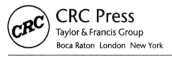

CRC Press
Taylor & Francis Group
Boca Raton London New York

CRC Press is an imprint of the
Taylor & Francis Group, an **informa** business

Designed cover image: Getty Images

First edition published 2025
by CRC Press
2385 NW Executive Center Drive, Suite 320, Boca Raton, FL 33431

and by CRC Press
4 Park Square, Milton Park, Abingdon, Oxon, OX14 4RN

CRC Press is an imprint of Taylor & Francis Group, LLC

© 2025 selection and editorial matter, Mary Collins; individual chapters, the contributors

ISBN: 978-1-032-46043-7 (hbk)
ISBN: 978-1-032-46041-3 (pbk)
ISBN: 978-1-003-37982-9 (ebk)

DOI: 10.1201/9781003379829

Typeset in Caslon
by KnowledgeWorks Global Ltd.

Contents

Foreword

As Head of the Dental School, a former Dean, Chair of Dental Education, Head of Programme, and a practising dentist for 39 years, I have often witnessed the profound positive impact Emotional Intelligence (EQ) can have on the quality of patient care delivered by the dental profession.

Dentistry is so much more than the dental professionals producing excellent clinical work for their patients. Patients' needs and expectations are in fact complex and comprehensive, and the carpentry on its own rings hollow without the quality of overall patient care going hand-in-hand. In fact, EQ plays a pivotal role in helping to establish trust and fostering patient satisfaction, building successful professional relationships between the dentist and the patient.

I am delighted to introduce you to *Emotional Intelligence in Dentistry: "Open Wide" – The Five Critical Skills to Take Dentists from Good to Great*, superbly written and presented by Dr Mary Collins from RCSI Centre of Positive Health Sciences, in collaboration a wonderful team of experts. It is a comprehensive, authoritative, and practical guide for every dentist and dental professional on EQ, from the most recently qualified to the most experienced colleagues alike.

Superbly presenting their research crystallising their vast expertise and experience, the authors have brilliantly illustrated the five key components in EQ in this book, namely, self-knowing, self-control, empathy, self-actualisation, and relationship skills. It instils a common sense, self-aware, refreshing and knowledge-based approach which reflects what practitioners can and should do to develop and retain their EQ.

What is most compelling about EQ is the emphasis on self-knowing. The journey undertaken by dental professionals to develop and maintain skills is continuous. By nurturing one's own EQ, dental professionals enrich competence, professionalism and personal lives. This book inspires you to offer the best patient care and professional satisfaction.

I thoroughly commend Mary, Martyn, Jason, and their colleagues. By integrating EQ into clinical dentistry, they empower and enrich the dental profession. I have no doubt that this book shall become an indispensable text for years to come, shaping the future of dentistry.

Grasp its wisdom, dive in and enjoy. Let *Emotional Intelligence in Dentistry: "Open Wide" – The Five Critical Skills to Take Dentists from Good to Great* empower you to enrich the lives of those you serve in clinical practice.

Professor Albert Leung
BDS LLM MA PhD FGDSRCS FDSRCS FDSRCPSG FFGDP FHEA
Head of School of Dentistry
Royal College of Surgeons in Ireland
Dublin, Ireland

Preface and Acknowledgements

For the last decade, I have had the privilege of working with healthcare leaders globally as part of my role in the Royal College of Surgeons Ireland (RCSI). A key part of this work is to support these healthcare professionals to develop their leadership capability. Leadership can often be viewed as an ambiguous ambition, lacking in definition and structure. In particular, there is a challenge working with exceptionally bright, talented "high IQ" professionals who seek evidence and science in everything they do. The work of pioneers in the Emotional Intelligence space such as Daniel Goleman and Reuven Bar-On and in more recent times, Dr Martyn Newman has been invaluable in bringing evidence and scientific rigour to this area.

In particular, the work of Dr Martyn Newman and the RocheMartin team in developing the Emotional Capital Report, a robust profile to assess and develop core emotional intelligence leadership competencies. I was struck in class recently when a bright, ambitious young trainee surgeon said to me, "Dr Collins – this is excellent, I can finally measure my leadership!"

Dentistry is a profession that impacts each of us at many points during our life span. The work of the profession is critical to our health and well-being. Sadly, the profession is also one where levels of depression and anxiety are common. My hope is that this book can support dentists at all career stages, from dental student to the later part of one's career in managing their emotions in a positive and constructive way.

I have focused on five core EQ competencies for this book: *self-knowing, self-control, empathy, relationship skills, and self-actualisation*. The rationale for this is that these are priority areas for development coming through from the initial research led by Dr Jason Atkinson and his team in Workforce Training and Education NHSE.

As the Royal College of Surgeons prepares to welcome its first undergraduate students in dentistry, I would like to acknowledge the wonderful leadership of our Head of School, Professor Albert Leung. Many thanks for sharing your insights and wisdom and writing the Foreword for this book.

My sincere thanks to Dr Martyn Newman for his immense support with this book. Martyn – you are leaving such a legacy for future generations of leaders in your pioneering work to make emotional intelligence a set of practical skills we all have the capability to develop.

I would also like to acknowledge the support of the wider RocheMartin team, especially the CEO, Guy Halfhead, and the Irish team, John and Maria Broderick, for their unwavering support of my work.

A special word of thanks to Dr Jason Atkinson and his team who pioneered important research with Foundation Year Dentists around EQ levels that was formative in the development of this book.

Writing this book has been an exciting, challenging journey into the world of dentistry. I am deeply grateful for each and every dentist who has shared their personal experiences and challenges with me in relation to the immense role of emotions in their work. In particular, I would like to acknowledge the dentists who contributed to each chapter of this book – Jason, Paul, Sally, Ian, Ciara, and Rory; you are all exemplary leaders in this important area. I am grateful for your insights, wisdom, kindness, and humour at all stages of the writing of this book!

To my dear colleagues in the RCSI Centre for Positive Health Sciences, in particular, our inspiring Founding Director, Prof Ciaran O'Boyle – thank you for your pioneering leadership and unwavering support for your team. You embody authentic leadership in so many ways.

Finally, my sincere thanks to Robert Peden, Senior Editor at CRC Press/Taylor & Francis, for his endless patience and support with this book.

This quote from Maya Angelou to me encapsulates the essence of emotional intelligence:

"People will forget what you said, people will forget what you did but people will never forget how you made them feel…."

My hope is that every dentist who picks up this book can find at least one practical insight to develop their emotional intelligence in some small way.

Mary Collins

Editor

Mary Collins is a Chartered Psychologist, author, and Senior Practitioner Coach (EMCC) who has been working in the Leadership Development/Talent Management field for over 20 years. Her current role as Senior Executive Development Specialist with RCSI Centre for Positive Health Sciences involves working with senior leaders in the healthcare sector to develop their management, coaching, and leadership capabilities through a range of executive development and academic programmes up to PhD level. Dr Collins also leads a successful business psychology practice working in a range of sectors in the area of talent and leadership development; prior to joining RCSI, she was Head of Talent and Learning for Deloitte Ireland for seven years.

Dr Collins is an Accredited Senior Professional Executive Coach and Coach Assessor with the European Coaching & Mentoring Council (EMCC) and became an Accredited Coach Supervisor in 2023 (ICCS). She is the current Co-chair of the Coaching Psychology Division of the Psychological Society of Ireland (PSI). In December 2019, she was one of 15 people awarded a "Coaching Hero Award" by the Minister of State for Higher Education from Kingstown College to mark her contribution to the coaching field in Ireland.

Dr Collins is passionate about leveraging the strengths of the Multigenerational Workplace and is a renowned key speaker on this topic. Her other research interests are Women in Leadership and Emotional Intelligence and Leadership. Her doctoral research has been published as part of the book *Managing Professionals & Other Smart People* in 2015. Her most recent book *Recruiting Talented Professionals* was published in May 2021.

Contributors

Jason Atkinson, is an Associate Postgraduate Dental Dean for Primary Care Dental Foundation training in Workforce Training and Education NHSE, working across the Yorkshire and Humber region. He oversees the education of all Dental Foundation Trainees and Dental Foundation Therapy Trainees on the DFT and DTFT programme and the two-year JDFCT programme. He has had broad experience across Foundation Training and Multi-Professional Education, having previously worked as a Training Program Director, Dental Tutor, Educational Supervisor, and a Vocational Trainee. In addition to his dental degree, he has gained a Postgraduate Certificate in Clinical Education and a Master's in Education, completing both programmes with a diverse range of healthcare professionals. As Associate Postgraduate Dean, Atkinson is fortunate and proud to work with a great team. This team – from Educational and Clinical Supervisors, DCPs, TPDs, and the many support staff that work in our training practices and for WTE NHSE – has one goal: to support and develop our trainees through a challenging and rewarding year. He recognises that these early years are crucial in developing skills and behaviours that will go on to shape the basis of a trainee's long-term success and happiness in general practice.

Sally Hanks qualified from Bristol Dental School in 1993 and has continued to work clinically in Primary Care Dentistry; in private, NHS and mixed practice, Community Dental Services, and as a civilian in the Armed Forces. She developed and honed her expertise looking after patients with a range of additional needs, including the use of hypnosis and other non-pharmacological anxiety and behaviour management techniques. Her academic career began as a Clinical Supervisor and Lecturer in Restorative Dentistry in 2008, and she is now a Professor of Primary Care Dentistry, Principal Fellow of Advance HE, and Associate Dean of Education and Student Experience for the University of Plymouth's Faculty of Health, which includes six schools. A new model of Leadership in Primary Care Dental Practice was developed in her PhD, which highlighted the importance of EI and she is recognised nationally and internationally as an expert in personal and professional development and education.

Martyn Newman, PhD, is a Clinical Psychologist specialising in emotional intelligence (EQ) and mindfulness. He is the author of the bestselling book *Emotional Capitalists* and newly released *The Mindfulness Book*. And co-author of the Emotional Capital Report™, the global benchmark for measuring EQ and leadership performance. Newman received his PhD from the University of Sydney and holds an MA from GTU at the University of California, Berkeley; a Master of Psychology from Monash University, Melbourne; and a Doctor of Psychology from La Trobe University, Melbourne. He has held academic posts as Senior Lecturer at the University of East London, the School of Psychology at ACU National, and is currently Visiting Fellow for Leadership at Sheffield Business School, Sheffield Hallam University, and an Instructor in Mindfulness on the MBA programme, Sydney University. Atkinson's advice has been sought at the highest levels of leadership worldwide, including the likes of Sky, Deloitte, ExxonMobil, Mars, Network Rail and Quiksilver, Royal Bank of Scotland, and British Airways, among many others.

Paul O'Dwyer, UCC dental graduate (1997), is the National Group Clinical Advisor with Portman Dentex (Ireland). He is also Adjunct Faculty at the Royal College of Surgeons in Ireland (Graduate School of Healthcare Management), where he lectures on clinical leadership and management. With a previous 15 years of general dental practice, Dr O'Dwyer has spent the last 10 years in Senior Management roles across three National Dental Corporate Organisations as Clinical Director. His current doctoral studies with the SPHeRE Programme look at communication in dental surgery. He was recently elected a Fellow of the American College of Dentists (2022), appointed Board Member of the Dental Health Foundation (2023), and continues his term as European Trustee of the International Pierre Fauchard Academy.

Rory O'Reilly graduated dental science from Trinity College Dublin in 2015. After several years working between hospital and community settings, O'Reilly left clinical practice to pursue sport in a full-time capacity. It was through his sport of kayaking that he first encountered coaching psychology. Having experienced the benefits on a personal and performance level, he pursued diploma and master's level qualifications in the area, completing his thesis on the use of coaching as a support for clinician well-being in dentistry. Currently, he works in private practice in London. He has a passion for teaching and enjoys teaching opportunities helping colleagues to better understand their relationship with dentistry, to find the right balance, and to improve soft skills like communication and relationship management.

Ciara Scott is a Specialist Orthodontist with extensive experience working in public, private, and dental school settings. She was awarded her Fellowship by the Faculty of Dentistry, RCSI in 2005 and completed an MSc at RCSI Institute of Leadership. In addition to her clinical experience, Scott currently holds an Adjunct Faculty role at RCSI Graduate School of Healthcare Management. She is a past Honorary Editor of the *Journal of the Irish Dental Association* and past President of the Orthodontic Society of Ireland. Her interest in enhancing person-centred care led her to completing EMCC-accredited training in coaching for workplace well-being, a Professional Diploma in Positive Psychology and Health at RCSI, and into research. In 2022, she was awarded a Health Research Board Scholarship to join the SPHeRE Programme as a PhD Scholar at the RCSI Centre for Positive Health Sciences.

Ian Wilson qualified as a dental surgeon at Edinburgh University in 1987 and has had extensive subsequent experience in Primary Care: he is the Co-founder and Clinical Director of the Dental Training & Development charity Bredge2Aid. As an experienced Dental Foundation Training Educational Supervisor, he is currently a Training Program Director within the Primary Care context. Wilson also acts as Clinical Advisor for Rodericks Dental, providing professional and pastoral support for their Primary Care clinical teams. With regard to mentoring, he has trained and mentored clinical teams developing oral health services alongside the Tanzanian Primary Care system, supported Dental Foundation trainees and peers as an ILM accredited coach/mentor, been RocheMartin-certified as an ECR Coach in Emotional Intelligence, and is an Associate with the Association of Coaching.

WHAT IS EMOTIONAL INTELLIGENCE IN PROFESSIONAL PRACTICE AND WHY DOES IT MATTER?

MARTYN NEWMAN

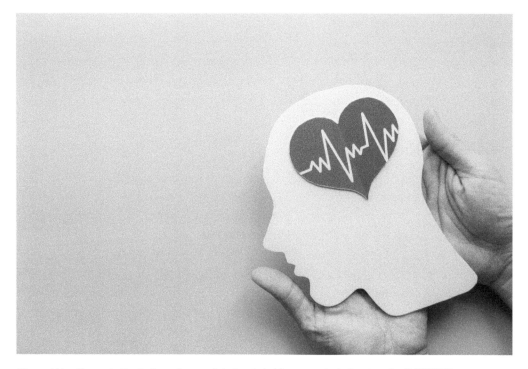

(*Source*: https://www.shutterstock.com/image-photo/hands-holding-paper-brain-heart-stroke-1815021524)

Twelve months after Andrew's graduation from dental school, our paths crossed for the first time. Nestled in an English country town, Andrew had established his practice, where he lived with his young family. Stepping into his clinic, I was greeted with genuine warmth. Andrew's eyes lit up as he noticed my slight accent, sparking a conversation that quickly evolved into an exchange of stories about our travels. Despite the half-full waiting room on that Friday afternoon, Andrew took a moment to reassure me about the wait time before attending to another patient.

As I settled into the waiting room, the receptionist handed me an intake questionnaire and offered me a drink. These small gestures, though seemingly insignificant, stood out to me, given my past experiences in National Health Service (NHS) dental practices. The attention to detail and the consideration for patients' comfort left a lasting impression.

DOI: 10.1201/9781003379829-1

Soon, a nurse named Georgie appeared and called my name. Her friendly demeanour put me at ease as she led me to the surgery. Curious about her background, I asked how long she'd been a dental nurse. Her enthusiastic response revealed that this was the first practice where she truly enjoyed her work. She recounted how meeting Andrew had reignited her passion for dentistry. Andrew had been able to describe the patient care that he wanted the practice to be known for; the treatments and procedures they wanted to specialise in, as well as the revenues he wanted to generate. "For the first time in my career I actually felt inspired," Georgie said. Andrew's vision for the practice, coupled with his commitment to building an inclusive team, had inspired her in ways she hadn't imagined.

Listening to Georgie's story, I couldn't help but reflect on my years of consulting with businesses. What she described – meaningful work, a supportive environment, a sense of belonging, and making a good living – echoed the core principles of successful organisations. It underscored the importance of what we often refer to as "soft skills" or emotional intelligence – or what I prefer to refer to as emotional capital.

Emotional Intelligence and Professional Practice

Emotional intelligence, or EQ, has long been recognised as a crucial factor in business success. However, its significance in professions like dentistry has only recently gained attention. Research suggests a positive correlation between a practitioner's EQ and treatment outcomes as well as patient satisfaction.

Rooted in the pioneering work of psychologists like Howard Gardner and John Mayer, emotional intelligence encompasses the ability to recognise, understand, and manage emotions effectively. Dan Goleman's seminal work *Emotional Intelligence* published in 1995 popularised the concept, emphasising its role in personal and professional effectiveness.

While IQ measures cognitive abilities, EQ complements it by addressing the emotional dimension of experience and its impact on perception, decision-making, and relationship-building. Together, they form a more holistic framework for understanding human intelligence and over the last two decades, research in neuroscience and psychology has highlighted the profound impact of EQ on various aspects of life. Individuals with high EQ demonstrate enhanced resilience, adaptability, and interpersonal skills, leading to improved job performance, higher job satisfaction, and personal well-being, all of which contribute to enhanced professional practice. Our own research over the last decade using the Emotional Capital Report (ECR) has validated these claims on a global scale.[1,2]

The Emotional Capital Model – Best Practice

There are a number of frameworks of emotional intelligence, but the most well-developed model for both measuring and developing emotional intelligence in a professional context is the Emotional Capital Model (**Figure 1.1**).[2] Divided into three

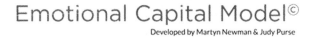

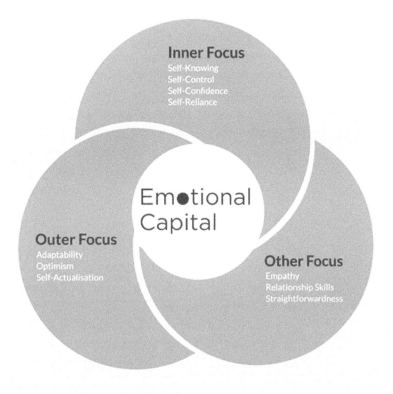

Figure 1.1   RocheMartin Emotional Capital Model of emotional intelligence. (See further Ref. [2].)

categories – inner focus, other focus, and outer focus – it highlights the importance of self-awareness, empathy, and adaptability in professional dental practice.

Inner focus encompasses a cluster of competencies crucial for understanding and managing personal emotional experience. It involves competencies such as self-knowing which is the capacity to recognise how feelings and emotions impact upon personal opinions, attitudes, and judgements, leading to greater self-awareness. But of course, the ability to notice emotions and manage them well also involves a second element of emotional intelligence, self-control. Self-control enables practitioners to manage stress, anxiety, and frustration effectively, both for themselves and their patients. By maintaining composure during challenging procedures, dental practitioners can ensure optimal patient care.

In addition, competencies such as self-confidence and self-reliance help shape patients' perceptions of the professional competence of a practitioner and influence treatment outcomes. Self-confident practitioners project competence, assurance, and credibility which are essential for building patient trust and rapport. Undeniably, in addition to the psychological aspects, developing self-confidence also involves mastering clinical skills, staying updated with advancements in the field, and continuing professional development.

Other focus emphasises empathy and relationship skills, essential for understanding and supporting patients' emotional experiences. Clear and empathetic communication fosters trust and mutual respect, enhancing patient satisfaction – an aspect of professional practice that apparently was critical to the success of Andrew's practice.

According to Andrew, "Dental care is inherently emotional and to succeed both professionally and from a treatment outcome point of view, dentists need the skills to communicate effectively with patients and support their emotional experience." Recognising the patient's particular experience and responding skilfully enables a practitioner to provide reassurance and establish a climate of psychological safety. And, research confirms that patients who feel understood, valued, and respected demonstrate greater patient compliance and ultimately report more positive treatment experiences.

A third competency, straightforwardness, involves conveying information clearly, accurately, and empathetically to patients. By fostering open dialogue, including involving the patient in co-diagnosis and treatment planning, as well as addressing patient concerns and providing realistic expectations, dental professionals can establish trust and mutual respect with their patients.

Outer focus involves competencies like adaptability, optimism, and self-actualisation, enabling practitioners to navigate change and embrace challenges. Optimism, for example, not only involves the capacity to sense opportunities and focus on the best possible outcomes of treatment, but it also establishes resilience in dealing with stress.

Young dentists entering the profession place a high priority on achieving a harmonious balance between their professional commitments and personal well-being. They acknowledge the demanding nature of their profession, marked by long hours, substantial patient loads, and the necessity to stay abreast of evolving practices. Nonetheless, they also value moments for self-care, leisure pursuits, and quality time spent with family and friends. Practice leaders who prioritise work-life equilibrium by providing flexible scheduling, ample time off, and supportive workplace policies are better positioned to attract and retain highly motivated professionals.

Dental School Training

Dental school training quite naturally focuses on academic and clinical achievements, often neglecting the development of emotional intelligence. Young graduates, like Andrew, may find themselves unprepared for the communication challenges and pressures of professional practice. Indeed, Andrew later confirmed to me, he felt completely ill-equipped to manage the intense pressure that working within the constraints that the NHS model had involved. The strain of having to meet the requirements to deliver an increasing number of units of dental activity had affected his ability to deliver the clinical standards he was committed to upon graduation. This experience had left him feeling demoralised.

Of course, traditionally, students like Andrew were not accepted into dental school based on their personal skills or emotional intelligence. By contrast, the entrance process focussed exclusively on their academic results based on their IQ rather than EQ. As a consequence, young graduates often step into the world of professional practice unprepared for the communication challenges of delivering high-quality patient care – including treatment plans, leading strong practice teams, and managing personal stress. These challenges, together with the strain of meeting NHS delivery requirements, lead many young graduate dentists such as Andrew to adopt a mixed-model practice that combines a private practice model with the NHS model.

Given the economic and social forces driving the NHS dental service and the challenges of modern practice, the stresses on the profession and individual dentists are only expected to increase. This is likely to lead many more clinicians either to adopt mixed-model practices like Andrew or leave the NHS altogether.

Conclusion – An Optimistic Future

Andrew's experience underscores the importance of incorporating the value of emotional intelligence into the training and preparation of dental practitioners. Clearly, clinical skills are of utmost importance, but it was Andrew's emotional and social competencies that had set his practice apart. By integrating emotional intelligence training into dental education and practice, we can foster a culture of excellence that emphasises enhanced patient communication, incorporating co-diagnostic models, verbal treatment plans, and enhanced standards of patient care.

I left Andrew's clinic that day not only satisfied with the treatment plan we'd agreed on together, but feeling more optimistic for the future of dentistry in the UK in general. If the dental profession is able to recruit and train more dentists like Andrew, equipping them with the skills of emotional intelligence, we could expect to see a lift in treatment outcomes, increased patient satisfaction, and a more rewarding career pathway that retains young professionals in the profession. Investing in the development of emotional intelligence not only benefits young dentists but also strengthens the future of the profession.

References

1. Newman M, Purse J, Smith K, Broderick J. Assessing Emotional Intelligence in Leaders and Organisations: Reliability and Validity of the Emotional Capital Report (ECR), Austral J Organisational Psychol, 2015;8: e6.
2. Newman M, Purse J. Technical Manual – The Emotional Capital Report, RocheMartin Pty Ltd., 2007.

WHY IS EMOTIONAL INTELLIGENCE SO CRITICAL FOR TODAY'S DENTIST?

MARY COLLINS

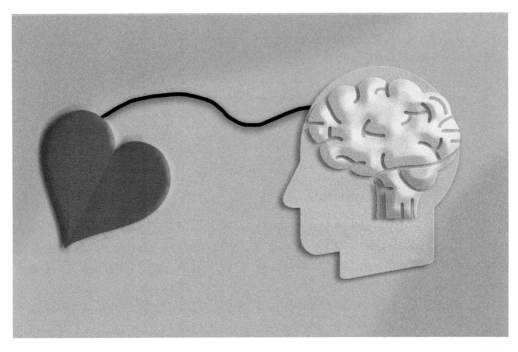

(*Source*: https://www.gettyimages.co.uk/detail/photo/brain-and-red-heart-connected-emotional-royalty-free-image/13315 65829?adppopup=true)

Introduction

Daniel Goleman, widely regarded as the 'Father of Emotional Intelligence' describes how crucial emotional intelligence (EI) is for our growth and profession in life:

> If your emotional abilities aren't in hand, if you don't have self-awareness, if you are not able to manage your distressing emotions, if you can't have empathy and have effective relationships, then no matter how smart you are, you are not going to get very far.

(Goleman, 2006)

EI is a critical area to develop for a successful career in dentistry. In a profession synonymous with high levels of stress, depression, and anxiety, the ability to be aware

DOI: 10.1201/9781003379829-2

of and manage emotions in oneself and in others is crucial to leading a successful and fulfilling career.

This chapter will explore the following topics:

- Challenges facing today's dental professional
- The role of EQ at every stage of the dental career
- Creating competitive advantage
- EQ as an imperative for the successful future of dentistry
- A case study of EQ research in postgraduate dental training

Challenges Facing Today's Dentists

Today's dentists navigate a complex landscape marked by rapid technological advancements, evolving patient expectations, costs of practice management, stress and mental health issues, regulatory and legal pressures, and a growing focus on environmental sustainability among many others. These multifaceted challenges require not only clinical expertise but also proficiency in business management, technology, and interpersonal communication.

Technological Advancements

Keeping pace with innovation is both an opportunity and a challenge. From digital impressions and CAD/CAM restorations to AI-driven diagnostic tools, technological advancements promise improved patient care and operational efficiency. However, as Schwendicke et al. (2020) point out, staying abreast of and proficient in these technologies demands continuous learning and significant financial investment.

Evolving Patient Expectations

Today's patients are more informed and empowered than ever before, often arriving at the dentist's office with expectations shaped by extensive online research or social media. While an informed patient base can facilitate engagement and compliance, it also poses challenges. Dentists must navigate misconceptions and misinformation, manage expectations regarding treatment outcomes, and communicate complex information in an accessible manner. Additionally, the increasing demand for cosmetic dentistry and aesthetic treatments requires dentists to balance patient desires with clinical considerations and ethical practices.

Gen Z patients are often described as 'digital natives' as they have grown up in the smartphone era, this has created an expectation for tech-enabled communications and also a demand for 'instant gratification' for requests, procedures, and so on. Dentists need to flex and adapt their approach for the Gen Z patient and also team members.

Costs of Practice Management

Running a dental practice involves significant overheads, from equipment and supplies to staffing and compliance costs. Private practices have additional financial pressures, including the complexities of navigating dental insurance policies and reimbursement rates that affect practice revenue and patient care affordability.

The attraction and retention of suitably qualified, motivated dental professionals at all levels remain a constant challenge in a tight labour market globally.

Stress and Mental Health Issues

The demanding nature of dental practice, compounded by business management pressures, can lead to high levels of stress and burnout. The dental profession is inherently stressful, characterised by high-performance expectations, demanding work schedules, and the emotional toll of patient care. Dentists must manage their own stress and well-being while providing compassionate care to patients who may be anxious or fearful. The risk of burnout is significant, with potential consequences for mental health, job satisfaction, and patient care quality.

Myers and Myers (2004) bring attention to this issue, highlighting the implications for practitioners' well-being. Indirect health issues like headaches, backache, and trouble sleeping for dentists are highlighted in this study.

Creating a sustainable work-life balance, seeking support through professional networks, and employing stress management strategies are essential for maintaining resilience in the face of these demands.

Regulatory and Legal Pressures

Dentists must adhere to a growing body of regulations related to patient privacy, data security, and health and safety standards. Moreover, the fear of legal action from dissatisfied patients can significantly impact stress levels and clinical decision-making.

Environmental Sustainability

The environmental impact of dental practices, particularly concerning waste management and energy use, is becoming an area of concern. Duane et al. (2019) emphasise the importance of adopting sustainable practices, a challenge that is increasingly expected by patients and society.

Navigating the complexities of modern dental practice requires a holistic approach that extends beyond clinical care. Today's dentists must engage in continuous professional development, embrace new technologies, adapt to changing patient expectations, manage their practices efficiently, and prioritise their well-being. By addressing these challenges head-on, dental professionals can continue to provide high-quality care, meet their patients' evolving needs, and ensure the sustainability of their practices in a rapidly changing healthcare landscape.

Role of Emotional Intelligence at Each Stage of the Dental Career

The role of EI (EQ) in dentistry is pivotal across all stages of a dentist's career, from dental school to retirement. EQ, a term popularised by psychologist Daniel Goleman, encompasses the ability to recognise, understand, manage, and use one's own emotions positively to relieve stress, communicate effectively, empathise with others, overcome challenges, and defuse conflict. In dentistry, where interactions with patients, staff, and colleagues are integral to everyday practice, EQ is invaluable for ensuring effective communication, building strong relationships, and fostering a supportive work environment.

Dental School

At this foundational stage, dental students must navigate the pressures of rigorous academic and clinical training while also beginning to interact with patients. Developing EI during these formative years can enhance learning experiences and foster better patient interactions. For instance, understanding and managing one's emotions can help students cope with the stress of exams and clinical performance, preventing burnout. Furthermore, empathetic communication skills are crucial for building trust with patients, even in a learning environment. Shapiro et al. (2004) emphasise the importance of incorporating EI development into medical education, noting its positive impact on professional competency and patient care.

Early Career

As new dentists transition into professional practice, they encounter the challenges of establishing themselves, building a patient base, and often managing a dental team. High EQ is critical during this stage for several reasons. Effective communication and empathy can greatly enhance patient satisfaction and loyalty, key factors in growing a successful practice. Additionally, the ability to manage one's emotions and understand those of colleagues can help navigate the dynamics of a dental team, fostering a positive and productive work environment. Goleman (1998) highlights that leaders with high EQ are more effective, as they can inspire and motivate their team, manage stress and conflict, and create an environment of cooperation and respect.

Mid-Career

Mid-career dentists often take on more significant leadership roles within their practices or the broader dental community, face complex clinical cases, and must keep pace with advancements in dental technology and procedures. At this stage, EQ contributes to leadership effectiveness, decision-making, and the continuous adaptation to change. High EQ enables dentists to lead by example, mentor younger colleagues, and navigate the stresses associated with professional growth and the evolution of their practice. This is also the time frame when dentists can typically be juggling work and family life, it is important to have good emotional regulation and stress management habits developed. Stein and Book (2011) argue that EI is a key factor in successful leadership and professional development.

Late Career

In the later stages of their careers, dentists might focus on legacy-building, such as mentoring new dentists, contributing to community health initiatives, or engaging in professional advocacy. EQ plays a significant role in these activities, facilitating meaningful connections, inspiring and guiding others, and navigating the emotional aspects of transitioning towards retirement. At this stage, the reflective component of EQ, including understanding and valuing the emotional journey of one's career, enriches the experience of passing on knowledge and contributing to the profession's future. According to Goleman et al. (2002), emotionally intelligent leaders can leave a lasting positive impact on their profession and community by fostering an environment of growth, empathy, and resilience.

Across the dental career spectrum, EQ is a critical factor in personal development, patient care, and professional success. From the anxiety of dental school to the challenges of practice management and the satisfaction of mentorship in later years, EQ provides the tools for dentists to manage their emotions, understand those of others, and navigate the complex interpersonal dynamics of the dental profession. Developing and nurturing EQ can lead to more rewarding career experiences, improved patient outcomes, and a positive workplace culture.

EI is not just an add-on to clinical skills; it is an integral component of a dentist's professional toolkit, essential for achieving excellence and fulfilment in their career.

EQ as a Competitive Advantage in Dentistry

Having high EI (EQ) provides a competitive advantage to dentists in many ways, impacting everything from self-leadership, patient care, practice management, and team dynamics. EI encompasses the ability to recognise, understand, manage, and use one's own emotions in positive ways to relieve stress, communicate effectively, empathise with others, overcome challenges, and defuse conflict. In the competitive landscape of dental care, where technical skills are given, EQ emerges as a critical differentiator that can elevate a dentist's practice from good to great. There follows a breakdown of some of the key differentiators for dentists high in EQ.

Enhancing Patient Satisfaction and Loyalty

High EQ enables dentists to better understand and respond to their patients' emotions, fostering a sense of trust and comfort. This empathetic approach can significantly improve patient satisfaction, an essential factor in building patient loyalty and generating positive word-of-mouth referrals. Cloninger and Cloninger (2011) emphasise that healthcare professionals with high EQ can create more meaningful patient interactions, leading to higher satisfaction rates. In the dental setting, where anxiety and fear are common, the ability to soothe, empathise, and communicate effectively can set a dentist apart from their peers.

Positive Work Environment

A successful dental practice is founded on a strong team. Dentists with high EQ possess leadership skills that inspire and motivate staff, foster a positive work environment, and effectively manage conflicts, contributing to improved team dynamics and staff retention. Stein and Book (2011) highlight that emotionally intelligent leaders are more successful in retaining their employees by creating a supportive and engaging workplace. High staff retention not only reduces recruitment and training costs but also contributes to a consistent, high-quality patient experience, and a more positive workplace culture.

Better Decision-Making

EI contributes to better decision-making by allowing dentists to manage their emotions and stress effectively, leading to clearer thinking and more rational decision-making. Dentists high in EQ, respond instead of react to challenging situations. This aspect of EQ is crucial when facing challenging clinical decisions, managing the business aspects of a practice, or navigating complex patient interactions. As we have seen above, according to Goleman et al. (2002) leaders with high EQ are better equipped to make informed, balanced decisions that consider both logical analysis and emotional insights.

Adaptability and Resilience

The dental profession, like all healthcare fields, is subject to constant change, whether due to technological advancements, regulatory changes, or shifts in patient expectations. Dentists with high EQ are more adaptable and resilient, traits essential for flourishing in a rapidly evolving landscape. They can navigate change more effectively, maintaining a positive attitude and an openness to new approaches. Mayer and Salovey (1997), who first coined the term 'emotional intelligence,' note that a key component of EI is the ability to manage emotions in ways that promote emotional and intellectual growth.

Building a Strong Practice Brand

A dentist's personal brand and the brand of their practice are increasingly important in a crowded marketplace. Dentists with high EQ can authentically connect with patients, staff, and the community, creating a strong, positive brand that attracts and retains patients and staff alike. This emotional connection can differentiate a dental practice in a competitive market, where patients are looking for providers who not only offer technical expertise but also genuinely care about their well-being.

In a profession where technical excellence is expected, EI offers a competitive edge that can make a significant difference in a dentist's success. From enhancing patient satisfaction and loyalty to improving team dynamics, facilitating better decision-making, enhancing adaptability, and building a strong practice brand, the benefits of high EQ are multifaceted. As the dental industry continues to evolve, the importance of EI will only grow, strengthening its role as a critical factor in achieving professional excellence and competitive advantage.

EQ and the Future of Dentistry

EI is becoming increasingly recognised as a critical component for the future of dentistry. This recognition comes at a time when the profession faces rapid changes in patient needs, heightened stress levels among dental professionals, and a broader understanding of the dentist's role beyond mere clinical expertise. EI, the ability to perceive, use, understand, and manage emotions, is pivotal in navigating these changes. Its importance is magnified by the shifting landscape of healthcare, where patient-centred care, professional well-being, and enhanced human skills are at the forefront.

Changing Patient Needs and Expectations

The landscape of patient needs and expectations in dentistry is evolving. Today's patients are more informed, empowered, and demanding than ever before. They seek not only high-quality clinical care but also a compassionate, empathetic approach from their healthcare providers. This shift towards patient-centred care places a premium on dentists' ability to understand and respond to the emotional and psychological needs of their patients.

EI enables dentists to excel in this environment. Dentists with high EQ are adept at reading their patients' emotions, leading to better communication and stronger patient-practitioner relationships. By empathising with patients, emotionally intelligent dentists can alleviate fears and anxieties, enhancing patient compliance and satisfaction. This empathetic approach is not just 'a nice to have' – it is essential for meeting modern patient expectations and fostering a loyal patient base.

Moreover, the increasing demand for cosmetic and aesthetic dental services further underscores the importance of EQ. These services often involve complex emotional motivations and expectations, requiring dentists to navigate sensitive discussions about self-image and aesthetics with tact and empathy.

Stress Management and Professional Well-Being

Dentistry is inherently a high-stress profession, characterised by demanding work schedules, complex patient interactions, and the need for precision in clinical procedures. The impact of chronic stress on dental professionals can be profound, leading to burnout, decreased job satisfaction, and even compromised patient care.

EI plays a crucial role in managing these stress levels. Self-awareness, a core component of EQ, enables dentists to recognise the early signs of stress and burnout, allowing them to take proactive steps to manage their well-being. Strategies may include seeking support, implementing work-life balance practices, and engaging in mindfulness or stress-reduction techniques.

Furthermore, EQ encompasses self-regulation, empowering dentists to control or redirect their disruptive emotions and impulses. This ability to manage emotions effectively is crucial in high-pressure situations, ensuring that stress does not negatively impact decision-making or patient care.

The Evolving Role of Dentists: Beyond Clinical Skills

The role of dentists is expanding beyond the confines of traditional clinical tasks. Today's dentists are leaders, communicators, educators, and advocates for oral health. This expanded role demands a comprehensive skill set that includes, and perhaps prioritises, human skills or 'soft skills' (which are actually the 'hardest of hard skills!'), such as communication, leadership, empathy, and adaptability – skills that are all core elements of EI.

Leadership is a particularly relevant aspect of the changing role of dentists. As leaders of their practices, dentists must inspire and motivate their teams, manage conflicts, and foster a positive workplace culture. EI is critical for these leadership tasks, enabling dentists to understand and influence the emotions of others effectively.

Moreover, as educators and advocates for oral health, dentists with high EQ can communicate more effectively, tailoring their messages to the emotional and informational needs of their audience. This ability is essential for promoting oral health, influencing healthy behaviours, and engaging with the community on public health initiatives.

The importance of EI in the future of dentistry cannot be overstated. As patient needs and expectations evolve towards a more holistic, patient-centred approach, dentists must be able to understand and empathise with their patients on a deeper level. The increasing stress levels within the profession call for a greater focus on self-awareness and self-regulation, ensuring that dentists can maintain their well-being and provide the best possible care. Finally, the expanding role of dentists in society demands a broader set of human skills, all of which are encompassed by EI.

Investing in the development of EI is not just beneficial; it is essential for dentists who wish to succeed in the rapidly changing landscape of healthcare. As the profession continues to evolve, those who prioritise EQ will find themselves better equipped to meet the challenges and opportunities of the future, ensuring a thriving practice and a fulfilling career in dentistry.

DENTAL PRACTITIONER PERSPECTIVE

JASON ATKINSON

Emotional Intelligence in the Early Years of Postgraduate Training Programmes

'Can you teach empathy?' was the final question fired at me during an interview I had at the start of my journey in dental education, nearly 30 years ago. I was applying to become a 'trainer' or as it is now classified an educational supervisor (ES) for newly qualified dentists (foundation dentists [FDs]), entering a postgraduate training and development programme; Dental Foundation Training (DFT). Like many prospective trainers at that time, my focus was on supporting clinical skills; influenced as is the case today, by a growing discourse on the clinical experience and readiness for newly qualified dentists to enter the dental workplace. The clinical focus on DFT is quite rightly highly relevant and important. For many new graduates, clinical skills are however a relatively straightforward area to develop and teach further, using recognised and established pathways that encompass simulation, observation, and experiential learning, supported by feedback from their assigned in practice educational supervisor. However, applying this developmental pathway to other non-technical skills and behaviours, such as empathy, communication or resilience can be problematic, not least due to in part that underlying attitudes and skills to non-technical behaviours, can often be hidden or masked by dental professionals, resulting in challenges for educational supervisors and the DFT programme to both identify, measure and support development. A renewed focus on factors that support performance as a dentist in the workplace have recognised the interplay other essential skills and behaviours have. These additional non-technical skills and behaviours have been grouped under additional Domains by both the governing body of dentistry in the UK, the General Dental Council (GDC), and are key components of the DFT curriculum, the Domains fall under three main areas: communication, management, and leadership, and professionalism. I have often reflected on the challenges in supporting the non-technical Domains, both personally and professionally over the intervening years. As my own involvement, knowledge, and experience of education have increased, I have challenged personal perspectives and biases on what 'teaching' can and should encompass. With an increased focus on personalised learner-centric education and teaching, colleagues and myself in Yorkshire and Humber have focused recently on an exploration and integration of an EI programme for FDs; in the hope to answer a fundamental question:

> How can our DFT program improve with the identification, support and development of essential non-technical skills and behaviours for the benefit of Foundation Dentists, patients and dental teams that are under our educational stewardship?

DOI: 10.1201/9781003379829-3

15

The Dental Foundation Training (DFT) programmes in England, Wales, and Northern Ireland (Dental Vocational Training in Scotland), are designed to support recent graduates, at the start of their careers in primary care dentistry. Over 95% of recent graduates enter the programme within two years of qualification and become FDs being assigned to a quality-managed NHS Primary Care Dental Training Practice and ES, who works within that practice as a dentist. The ES is carefully selected to ensure they have the necessary skills and behaviours to act as a role model, mentor, and clinical teacher. The DFT programme provides opportunities to gain clinical experience, with appropriate supervision available, within authentic workplace conditions; with supplemental educational support and quality management of the programmes being provided by local 'deaneries' across the UK.

Most FDs complete the DFT programme after one year, with a smaller proportion being placed in a more comprehensive two-year scheme, where they gain concurrent experience in both an NHS dental practice and secondary care, hospital-based programmes. From a primary dental care perspective, the aim of both the one- and two-year programmes is to provide, under satisfactory completion, confirmation, and assurance that the FD is capable of working independently as a 'safe' NHS General Dental Practitioner (GDP), within the NHS Primary Care Dental Services in the UK.

The role of an NHS GDP encompasses a complex and often conflicting synergy of both the clinical technical domains and non-technical domains, where they are expected to concurrently meet and balance personal human challenges in life with the expectations of patients, the NHS system, regulatory bodies and the varied interpersonal demands of the workplace culture and environment. While the synergy of the domains a dentist is expected to work within, can be expressed, viewed, and are demonstrated holistically in the workplace through observable activities and interactions, it is challenging to understand, influence and support the hidden beliefs, emotions and attitudes that underpin these complex interactions. While it is true that both technical and non-technical skills and behaviours are of equal importance, from a patient's perspective it is arguably the non-technical skills that provide the most reassurance that they are being listened to and treated safely and appropriately. Increasing evidence has highlighted the consequences should a dentist struggle to resolve the varying demands that dental practice places them under, with many of complaints that escalate to either litigation or professional sanctions stemming from apparent deficiencies within the 'non-technical' domains. Working within a 'target'-based NHS Dental System, that does not currently positively recognise the quality of care that is provided, in addition, to the many regulatory, financial, and interpersonal challenges of practice working and ownership, which some dentists choose to enter; it is not surprising that there appears to be an increase in dentists who experience significant stress, depression, and burnout within the profession as a whole.

On entering DFT programmes, all FDs will be fully registered dental professionals with GDC, being expected to work under the same regulatory standards as their more experienced dental colleagues. Although working under supervision and within a supportive environment; for many FDs this will be the first time they have entered a workplace environment where they have significant leadership responsibilities, equally many will have left school and entered undergraduate training without any experience of working within a team-based culture with a common quality-driven objective.

The FD will be seeing patients within the first few weeks of training, patients will rightly have expectations on the quality of care and interactions they receive from the dentists they see, regardless of their current level of experience. Although supportive, the dental team within the training workplace will also expect certain behaviours and skills from the FD they are supporting. Although FDs are somewhat protected from the NHS target-driven system that all NHS GDPs subsequently work under, the other demands and expectations a GDP will experience are still present. Some FDs will face, potentially for the first time in their lives, complaints or challenges from patients or colleagues; coupled with inexperience, these situations are challenging and in stark contrast to the more directed and protected environment of an undergraduate dental school.

Over the past 10 years, anecdotally, myself and colleagues across all DFT programmes in the UK, have routinely experienced FDs struggling with the pressures of their role and the increased responsibilities this places them under. While many FDs cope incredibly well and quickly adapt to the new workplace and leadership role they have assumed, a significant number struggle with managing both integration into an established dental team and the expectations that patients, the GDC, the DFT programme, and established practice teams expect. This often manifests with the FD expressing feelings of not fitting in within a team, difficulties dealing with conflict, expressions of feeling inadequate, difficulties coping and effectively managing stressful situations within the workplace, dealing with varying patient complaints, rejection, concerns, or failure and importantly, for some, the potential to go on and develop significant mental health concerns, which can often result in time off from work and occasionally targeted professional health and mental well-being support.

It is important to remember that the resilience an FD possesses to manage and cope with these common workplace challenges and experiences, does not appear to be directly linked to the quantitative amount of prior undergraduate clinical experience an FD brings with them to the workplace. The role that EI has on the self-management of these common experiences is clear in my view, but up until relatively recently, no robust evidenced-based method of pre-emptive or reactive identification of competencies linked to EI have been available or introduced for FDs. Furthermore, without identification and appropriate evidenced-based support, it will be difficult to provide focused and tailored external support and development strategies for FDs.

A key quality management component of the DFT programme involves regular workplace-based assessments and feedback, designed to support and facilitate the development of both clinical and non-clinical skills and behaviours. The assessments are essential and provide strong evidence towards meeting the expected outcomes of the programme. A powerful formative educational assessment utilised in DFT involves anonymous multi-source feedback (MSF) from the team members working with the FD in practice as well as patient feedback. MSF has been demonstrated to be an effective assessment of non-technical skills, often highlighting areas for development. However, the learning plans from MSF often result in 'objectives' such as 'listen to the team more,' 'show more appreciation to colleagues' and 'you'll become more confident as you gain more experience.' While on a superficial level, these plans are specific with the outcomes being measurable through observation in the workplace, they assume that the FD possesses the necessary skills and insight to action improvements in a meaningful manner. Critically, observable improvements do not preclude an FD from artificially masking these behaviours through actions that may not be either genuine or reflective of a significant change in how an FD internalises and develops themselves. A lack of meaningful improvement in these EI critical areas may also crucially hamper an FD's progress within the DFT programme and subsequent satisfactory completion of the programme. Of equal importance, for FDs who fail to improve in non-technical skills, there is an increased likelihood of them experiencing a continuation of negative and stressful experiences within the workplace, that lead to an increased likelihood of patient complaints and litigation, conflict with team members, and mental health deterioration.

To help support FDs both develop insight and support growth with their own EI, and the important role it plays in supporting and developing non-technical skills, the Yorkshire and Humber Postgraduate region has piloted over three years an EI programme for DFT. Starting with the 2021/2022 cohort of FDs, the EI programme was facilitated through a globally recognised provider of EI training and support – RocheMartin. The EI programme RocheMartin utilises is based on the work of Professor Martyn Newman who developed a strong evidence-based self-assessment of EI, called the Emotional Capital Report (ECR; Newman and Purse, 2007) and a certified coaching approach to help enable both the identification and development of EI among individuals. Critically, the research evidence demonstrates that EI is not an intransigent fixed attribute for individuals, but can be developed and supported, through an evidence-based approach. The ECR and EI programme defines and relates to 10 core competencies of EI, linked to inner or 'self'-competencies, other or 'patient/colleagues' competencies, and 'outer' competencies, focused on both future career development/engagement, satisfaction, and professional progression (**Table 2.1**).

The EI programme in DFT, involved the completion of self-evaluation questionnaires (ECR) by FDs with the results being linked to a formative developmental programme of specific EI competency-focused workshops and 1:1 coaching through trained EI coaches, facilitated by access to self-help guides and resources for FDs.

We have found since this programme was launched for cohorts of approximately 96 trainees each year, there was a strong correlation between the results of the ECR FDs complete and independent identification of development opportunities highlighted through MSF or ES feedback and more encouragingly, self-directed development requests from the FDs themselves.

Although all EI competencies are important and are developed through coaching within the DFT programme, the following areas have particular significance in

Table 2.1 Focuses and Competencies

FOCUS	COMPETENCY
Inner (Self)	• Self-knowing • Self-control • Self-confidence • Self-reliance
Others (Colleagues/Patients)	• Empathy • Relationship skills • Straightforwardness
Outer	• Optimism • Self-actualisation • Adaptability

relation to frequent challenges an FD may experience within the workplace and the interactions they experience with colleagues and patients. A snapshot of the results for 96 FDs in the 2021/2022 cohort, demonstrates how an FDs inner focus on self-knowing and self-control, linked to a focus on others, through empathy and relationship-building, could support positive interactions in the workplace. Conversely, deficiencies in these very same areas can contribute to difficulties an FD has in managing interactions with patients and workplace colleagues, which as described are common areas of difficulties some FDs experience during DFT.

Self-Knowing and Self-Control (Inner Focus)

The foundations for forming positive relationships with patients and team members start with the FDs ability to have insight and awareness of their own emotional state and how to mitigate knee-jerk emotional reactions to challenging clinical situations. FDs can often face challenging or difficult clinical challenges, primarily due to a lack of clinical experience and contextual clinical knowledge on how best to approach a clinical scenario. Having awareness of your own emotional state, self-knowing, which could be affected by difficulties outside of the dental practice, provides an FD with an opportunity to analyse, rationalise, and mitigate these emotions in the clinical workplace. Equally important is the ability to mitigate primal emotions and practice self-control when faced with challenges. Gaining competency in these skills can help an FD appear or behave confident and in control of clinical situations, helping to reassure patients and allow space for critical analytical skills to develop, leading to displays of calm, reassuring, and confident behaviours in front of patients and the dental team. For some FDs, appearing less than confident with clinical decision-making and dealing with treatments that have not provided optimum results have been highlighted through the MSF assessment. If these emotions are translated into uncertainty in front of patients, or the FD becomes overly defensive, coupled with a potential to not display empathy, a patient could quickly lose trust in an FD-proposed treatment, or suggested resolution, leading to patients either asking to be seen by another dental professional, or in certain situations, raising a complaint; both of which further increase the stress and confidence an FD has in themselves.

For interactions with colleagues, having awareness and control of emotional reactions in the workplace can support positive interactions within the dental team, avoiding and mitigating escalation of potential conflict, helping the FD to diffuse situations and understand the role they play. Self-control and self-knowing competencies are especially important for FDs to develop further since they will have minimal previous workplace experience to draw upon. These skills are especially critical for the leadership journey FDs are undertaking, where they are expected to manage a team effectively and act as role models within that team.

Overall, the ECR results for self-knowing (**Figure 2.1**) demonstrated that most FDs had good levels of competence, highlighting that they should have a solid understanding and awareness of how their emotional state could affect decision-making and interactions with patients and colleagues. However, for self-control (**Figure 2.2**), a significant number of FDs potentially have difficulties in managing pressure and controlling emotional reactions. Coaches provided support for FDs in both areas, to help

Mean	100.78
Median	102
Mode	99
Standard Deviation	11.95

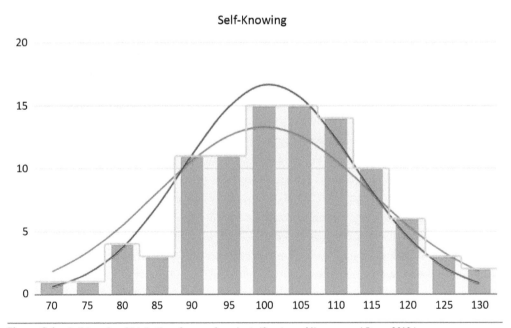

Figure 2.1   Self-knowing: Distribution of scores for cohort. (Courtesy of Newman and Purse 2018.)

Mean	94.16
Median	94
Mode	91
Standard Deviation	11.14

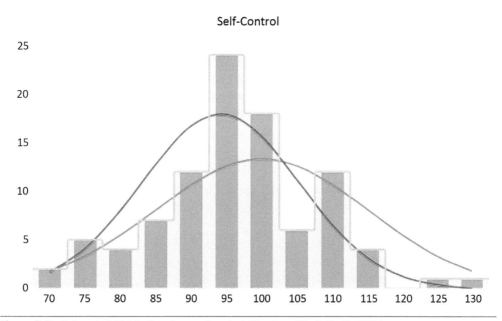

Figure 2.2   Self-control: Distribution of scores for cohort. (Courtesy of RocheMartin 2022.)

them to become aware of how their own emotions and a lack of control in naturally stressful situations could contribute to perceived erratic behaviours, impacting negatively on both their own stress levels and that of colleagues and patients. Importantly, good levels of competence in both these areas would support the development and ability to form healthy and productive relationships within the dental team.

Relationship skills are recognised as a separate competency within the ECR describing the ability for FDs to establish and maintain healthy professional relationships within the dental teams who are supporting them in the DFT programme. Both self-knowing and self-control have an influence on how relationships are maintained and nurtured. For this group, again most FDs displayed good levels of competence overall with developing and maintaining health relationships (**Figures 2.3** and **2.4**). These skills were again confirmed through analysis of the overall positive MSF feedback FDs received from teams for this cohort. However, the results also highlight a significant minority of FDs who may have difficulty in initiating and building relationships with team members, narrowing the potential scope for support received

Mean	101.15
Median	102
Mode	92
Standard Deviation	12.04

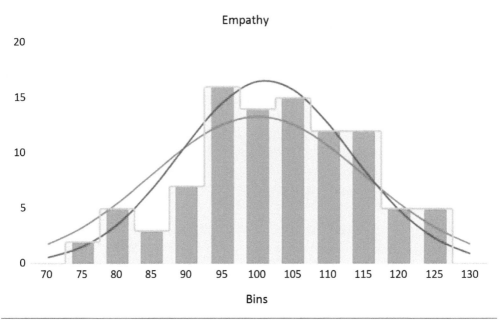

Figure 2.3 Empathy: Distribution of scores for cohort. (Courtesy of RocheMartin 2022.)

during the DFT programme. I am aware of FDs expressing feelings of isolation or loneliness when working in a team for the first time, which could lead to a decline in both the FD's own mental health and overall satisfaction with working as a dentist and the potential for this to adversely affect progress towards achieving the long-term goals of the DFT programme. The EI programme focused on practical advice that supports relationship-building, as this factor is critical for both effective teamwork and feelings of positive integration within an established dental team. An important component of building relationships with both colleagues and patients is empathy, the ability to understand the feelings of another.

Displaying authentic empathy for patients has been shown to be a significant factor in relation to reducing litigation claims and patient complaints that healthcare professionals may experience during their career. Empathy for team members and the effects an FD's actions and behaviours could have on forming relationships, is also important. Reassuringly for a profession that is patient-centred, most FDs possessed

Mean	102.65
Median	104
Mode	104
Standard Deviation	13.50

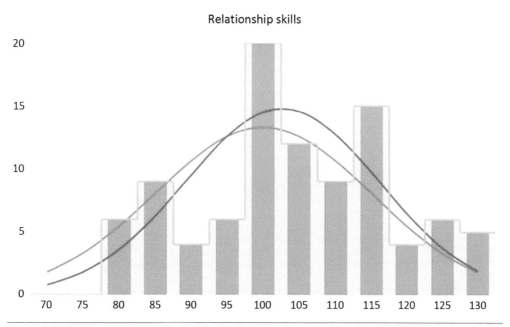

Figure 2.4   Relationship skills: Distribution of scores for cohort. (Courtesy of RocheMartin 2022.)

very good levels of empathy; however, a significant proportion, around a third had potential areas for development and growth in this area (**Figure 2.3**). Group coaching was provided that covered this area, with a particular focus on FDs who had low scores in this area or who had experienced a patient complaint through a perceived lack of communication, in particular relating to listening skills. Within DFT programmes there is time for this skill to be developed since the programme is crucially protected from the NHS target-driven narrative, affording more time for FDs to listen to patients and understand their expectations from the care they are seeking.

Finally, the importance of self-actualisation will be described for this cohort of FDs, and how recognising a balance between the sometimes-competing challenges of professional, personal, and financial demands influence long-term performance and overall well-being. Self-actualisation describes both the inner ability for FDs to find passion for the work that they do, as dentists and how that passion can be developed to influence themselves and others within the profession. Having passion for dentistry and demonstrating that within the workplace, through enthusiasm, quality improvement and a work ethic is contagious, positively influencing workplace cultures. Even at an early stage in an FD's career, the positive effect they can have on established workplace cultures should not be underestimated. I consistently receive overwhelming feedback from ESs and dental teams on the positive reinvigorating effect an FD can have on an established workplace culture, being one of the main reasons why they support and engage with the DFT programme. The ECR process has both highlighted this to FDs and the potential they can bring to the workplace, but also highlights to them the challenges that can affect this, balancing the challenges of personal and professional lives. Conversely, an FD who cannot find the energy to maintain this enthusiasm for their role, can lead to declines in both the performance of themselves and disillusionment within the dental team that is tasked with supporting them.

It would be reasonable to expect that FDs, at the very start of their careers have good levels of self-actualisation; for the majority, this is the case (**Figure 2.5**). Although FDs leave dental school with a high level of personal debt, the FD role is

Mean	96.65
Median	97
Mode	104
Standard Deviation	12.34

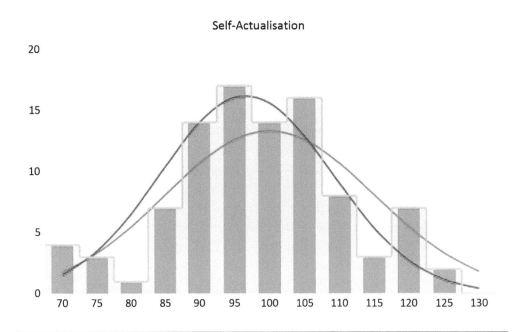

Figure 2.5 Self-actualisation: Distribution of scores for cohort. (Courtesy of RocheMartin 2022.)

salaried and provides some financial security. However, there will naturally be challenges and demands within their own personal lives and equally through a combination of relatively low experience with both treating patients and working in authentic workplace environments, challenges within their professional lives. Maintaining and developing this competency, both during DFT and beyond is critical in supporting resilience and well-being of the FD themselves and the positive effect they will have as future leaders in the profession. A significant proportion of FDs (approximately 25%) highlighted significant deficits in self-actualisation, through the ECR process. We have therefore been able to provide access to both self-help resources and where indicated, coaching to provide more tailored support for this group, with the hope we can positively influence this crucial aspect of EI, mitigating against potential disillusionment and adverse mental health consequences.

Overall, the work completed to date with EI development has provided a robust process of support and development for FDs in the Yorkshire and Humber DFT programme.

For the first time, the DFT faculty team have access to a methodology which both identifies and supports FD cohorts, with programmes of development that target critical skills and behaviours that are key components of holistic patient care, teamwork, and leadership. We have utilised the ECR through triangulating its results with workplace feedback and that of the FD themselves to provide 1:1 coaching, and provided the entire cohort with focused workshops on key elements that support the non-technical skill development so crucial for safe and effective patient care. Over the last three years, the feedback from FDs has been overwhelmingly positive, with a quote from an FD below, summarising the effect this has had:

> Whether working within the dental team or finding a work-life balance I've found the experience of coaching enlightening as it's helped me to understand myself. It's sparked changes in my personal and professional life and made me recognise certain strengths and weaknesses. I feel in a much stronger position to make use of my training and skills from university and I'm grateful for it.

Equally, our ESs have also noticed significant changes within the workplace, for FDs that have progressed through the EI programme.

For myself personally, I have answered a question that started my career in Dental Education, 'Can you teach Empathy?' in the context of what teaching should encompass, through a renewed focus on the individual and via the application of coaching with access to appropriate evidence-based resources, the answer is a resounding 'Yes!'

Acknowledgements

Introducing an emotional intelligence programme within Yorkshire and Humber Dental Foundation Training would not have been possible without the support of the entire team that enables continual quality improvements. This includes every member of the team: those working in our training locations, the managerial support team that helps to coordinate and support DFT, and the members of my own clinical team, who have consistently and enthusiastically understood why emotional intelligence is an important aspect of the support and teaching we provide to foundation dentists.

I would also like to thank and recognise the following colleagues, who were instrumental in introducing and supporting the programme at its inception:

- James Spencer, Postgraduate Dental Dean
- Ian Wilson, Training Program Director (Yorkshire and Humber) and EI Coach
- Anthony Kilcoyne, Training Program Director (Yorkshire and Humber) and EI Coach
- Guy Wells, CEO RocheMartin
- Dr Martyn Newman, Chairman, RocheMartin
- All educational supervisors, DFT programmes in Yorkshire and Humberside

References

Cloninger CR, Cloninger KM (2011) Person-centered therapeutics. *Int J Pers Cent Med*;1(1): 43–52.

Duane B, Harford S, Ramasubbu D, Stancliffe R, Pasdeki-Clewer E, Lomax R, Steinbach I (2019) Environmentally sustainable dentistry: A brief introduction to sustainable concepts within the dental practice. *Br Dent J*;226(4):292–295.

Goleman D (1998) *Working with Emotional Intelligence*. Bantam Books.

Goleman D (2006) *Emotional Intelligence: The Tenth Anniversary Edition*. Bantam Books.

Goleman D, Boyatzis R, McKee A (2002) *Primal Leadership: Learning to Lead with Emotional Intelligence*. Harvard Business School Press.

Mayer JD, Salovey P (1997) What is emotional intelligence? In Salovey P, Sluyter DJ, eds, *Emotional Development and Emotional Intelligence: Educational Implications*. Basic Books: 3–34.

Myers HL, Myers LB (2004) It's difficult being a dentist': Stress and health in the general dental practitioner. *Br Dent J*;197(2):89–93; discussion 83; quiz 100–1.

Newman M, Purse J (2018) *Emotional Intelligence Certification Workbook*. RocheMartin Pty Ltd.

Newman M, Purse J (2007) *Emotional Capital Report – Technical Manual*, Roche Martin Institute, Melbourne.

RocheMartin (2022) *The ECR and EQ Program for the 2021/22 FD Cohort*. RocheMartin Pty Ltd.

Schwendicke F, Samek W, Krois J (2020) Artificial intelligence in dentistry: Chances and challenges. *J Dent Res*;99(7):769–774.

Shapiro J, Morrison E, Boker J (2004) Teaching empathy to first year medical students: Evaluation of an elective literature and medicine course. *Educ Health*;17(1):73–84.

Stein SJ, Book HE (2011) *The EQ Edge: Emotional Intelligence and Your Success*, 3rd ed. Jossey-Bass.

3
EMOTIONAL INTELLIGENCE CRITICAL SKILL I

Self-Knowing

MARY COLLINS

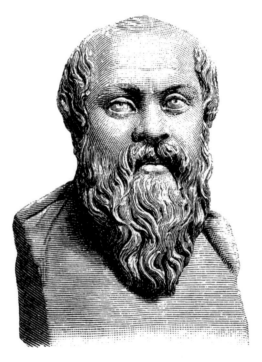

(*Source*: https://www.gettyimages.co.uk/detail/illustration/socrates-bust-royalty-free-illustration/1372384762?adppopup =true)

The ancient Greek philosopher Socrates is credited with saying "to know thyself is the beginning of wisdom." This quote describes the importance of self-awareness as the foundation for understanding the world around us and making wise decisions. It captures the essence of self-reflection and highlights that true insight begins with an inward journey of understanding one's own thoughts, emotions, and actions.

This chapter will focus on the foundational emotional intelligence (EI) competency of "self-knowing" covering the following topics:

- Defining self-knowing
- Why is self-knowing important in dentistry?
- How best to develop this area
- Dental practitioner perspective

DOI: 10.1201/9781003379829-4

What Is Self-Knowing

Self-knowing or self-awareness is one of the foundational competencies of all EI frameworks. Dr Martyn Newman, a renowned clinical psychologist and expert in EI and leadership, defines self-knowing in his Emotional Capital Report (ECR) as "the ability to recognise and understand your moods, emotions, and drives, as well as their effect on others." This definition emphasises the dual aspect of self-knowing: the internal understanding of oneself and the external awareness of the impact one's emotions have on others. According to Newman, self-awareness is not only about recognising and understanding one's emotional state but also about leveraging this awareness to guide decision-making, communication, and behaviour in a social context.

Self-knowing refers to an individual's awareness of their own emotions, strengths, weaknesses, values, and drivers. This competency is foundational because it influences how individuals perceive themselves and interact with others around them. Understanding the manifestations of high and low levels of self-knowing can provide insights into professional behaviour and personal development (**Table 3.1**).

Table 3.1   Self-Knowing: Behaviours of High and Low Levels in the Workplace

HIGH SELF-KNOWING BEHAVIOURS AT WORK	LOW SELF-KNOWING BEHAVIOURS AT WORK
When someone possesses a high level of self-knowing, we see the following characteristics in their behaviour and interactions:	When someone possesses a low level of self-knowing, we see the following characteristics in their behaviour and interactions:
1. *Personal insight*: Individuals with high self-knowing have a deep understanding of their emotional states, preferences, and drives. They recognise how their feelings can affect their thoughts and behaviours and understand their strengths and limitations.	1. *Lack of self-awareness*: People with low self-knowing may have a limited understanding of their emotions and how these emotions influence their behaviour. They might struggle to identify why they feel a certain way or how to address their feelings constructively.
2. *Emotional regulation*: These individuals can manage their feelings effectively as they understand their emotions well, even in stressful or challenging situations. They are less likely to react impulsively and more likely to respond in considered and constructive ways.	2. *Impulsive reactions*: With a lack of understanding of their emotional triggers, individuals are more likely to react impulsively to stress or provocation. This can lead to conflict and misunderstandings in professional and personal relationships.
3. *Authenticity*: High self-knowing leads to authenticity; individuals with high self-knowing tend to be more genuine to themselves in all circumstances. This authenticity fosters trust and credibility with colleagues, staff, and patients.	3. *Difficulty in stress management*: People with low self-knowing often find it challenging to manage stress effectively. They may be unaware of their stress signals and thus unable to employ coping strategies until they are overwhelmed.
4. *Effective communication*: Understanding their emotional state helps individuals communicate more clearly and effectively. They can express their needs, thoughts, and feelings in a way that is direct yet empathetic, enhancing interpersonal relationships.	4. *Impact on interpersonal relationships*: A lack of emotional self-awareness can hinder the ability to form and maintain healthy relationships. These individuals might struggle to empathise with others or communicate their needs and feelings clearly.
5. *Reflective learning*: Individuals with high self-knowing tend to be reflective learners. They possess the ability to accurately evaluate their own performance, identify areas that require improvement, and are receptive to receiving feedback. This quality supports continuous personal and professional development.	5. *Resistance to feedback*: Without a clear understanding of their strengths and development areas, individuals may be defensive about feedback. This resistance can limit personal growth and professional development.
6. *Resilience*: These people tend to have a strong sense of self. This can help navigate setbacks and challenges with a positive outlook. They perceive challenges as prospects for development, which enhances their capacity for resilience.	

High Self-Knowing

When someone possesses a high level of self-knowing, we see the following characteristics in their behaviour and interactions:

1. *Personal insight*: Individuals with high self-knowing have a deep understanding of their emotional states, preferences, and drives. They recognise how their feelings can affect their thoughts and behaviours and understand their strengths and limitations.

2. *Emotional regulation*: These individuals can manage their feelings effectively as they understand their emotions well, even in stressful or challenging situations. They are less likely to react impulsively and more likely to respond in considered, constructive ways.

3. *Authenticity*: High self-knowing leads to authenticity; individuals with high self-knowing tend to be more genuine to themselves in all circumstances. This authenticity fosters trust and credibility with colleagues, staff, and patients.

4. *Effective communication*: Understanding their emotional state helps individuals communicate more clearly and effectively. They can express their needs, thoughts, and feelings in a way that is direct yet empathetic, enhancing interpersonal relationships.

5. *Reflective learning*: Individuals with high self-knowing tend to be reflective learners. They possess the ability to accurately evaluate their own performance, identify areas that require improvement, and are receptive to receiving feedback. This quality supports continuous personal and professional development.

6. *Resilience*: These people tend to have a strong sense of self. This can help navigate setbacks and challenges with a positive outlook. They perceive challenges as prospects for development, which enhances their capacity for resilience.

Low Self-Knowing

When someone possesses a low level of self-knowing, we see the following characteristics in their behaviour and interactions:

1. *Lack of self-awareness*: People with low self-knowing may have a limited understanding of their emotions and how these emotions influence their behaviour. They might struggle to identify why they feel a certain way or how to address their feelings constructively.

2. *Impulsive reactions*: With a lack of understanding of their emotional triggers, individuals are more likely to react impulsively to stress or provocation. This can lead to conflict and misunderstandings in professional and personal relationships.

3. *Difficulty in stress management*: People with low self-knowing often find it challenging to manage stress effectively. They may be unaware of their stress signals and thus unable to employ coping strategies until they are overwhelmed.

4. *Impact on interpersonal relationships*: A lack of emotional self-awareness can hinder the ability to form and maintain healthy relationships. These

individuals might struggle to empathise with others or communicate their needs and feelings clearly.

5. *Resistance to feedback*: Without a clear understanding of their strengths and development areas, individuals may be defensive about feedback. This resistance can limit personal growth and professional development.

Importance of Self-Knowing in Dentistry

Self-knowing plays a critical role in shaping the professional practice and personal growth of dental professionals from the student stage right through to retirement. According to Dr Martyn Newman, a leading psychologist in the field of EI and leadership, self-knowing is defined in his ECR as "the ability to recognise, understand and manage one's own emotions and to be aware of the impact of those emotions on others and on oneself." This definition underscores the importance of self-awareness, emotional regulation, and the recognition of one's emotional influence on others, all of which are pivotal for effective communication, decision-making, and relationship-building in the context of dentistry.

Dentistry is a profession that demands a high degree of technical skill, social awareness, and emotional resilience – all of these areas are supported by high levels of self-knowing. Dentists and dental professionals frequently encounter patients experiencing anxiety, fear, and discomfort. The awareness and ability to understand and manage one's emotional responses is essential for creating a positive patient experience and for maintaining a compassionate and empathetic practice.

The main benefits to develop self-knowing are outlined below.

Enhanced Patient Care

Self-knowing supports dentists to better navigate the emotional aspects of patient care. As a result of understanding their own emotional triggers and responses, dentists can cultivate a more patient-centred approach that acknowledges and addresses the emotional needs and concerns of their patients. This empathetic engagement can lead to increased patient satisfaction, compliance, and overall better health outcomes. Studies have shown that EI, including self-knowing, correlates with more effective patient communication, improved care quality, and reduced levels of litigation.

Professionals who have developed a deep sense of self-knowing are better equipped to exhibit genuine empathy, as they are aware of their own emotional responses and can therefore more effectively tune into the emotions of others.

Empathy allows healthcare providers to connect with patients on a deeper level, genuinely understanding their experiences, fears, and hopes. A study by Babaii et al. (2021) underscores the link between provider empathy and patient satisfaction, indicating that empathetic care leads to better patient outcomes.

Improved Decision-Making

The high-pressure environment of a dental practice requires fast and effective decision-making. Self-knowing contributes to this by providing dentists with the emotional clarity needed to make informed decisions in a calm, composed way. When dentists are aware of their emotional states, they are less likely to be impacted by stress and more likely to approach clinical decisions with a balanced and rational perspective.

Dental professionals often face complex ethical dilemmas and must make decisions under pressure. A deep understanding of one's values and ethical principles, core aspects of self-knowing, is crucial in these moments. By reflecting on their own beliefs and emotional responses, professionals can navigate these challenging situations with integrity, aligning their actions with the best interests of their patients.

Stress Management and Resilience

A study published by Collin et al. (2019) found that nearly half of dentists experience job-related stress, with regulation and patient litigation being the most stressful factors.

A key component of self-knowing is the ability to recognise and manage one's emotions. This is essential for coping with the stresses inherent in the dental profession. Dentists face many daily challenges, from managing complex patient cases to navigating the complex dynamics of dental practice. Self-knowing can help in identifying stressors and emotional triggers. Awareness is the first stage in change, once aware of what these stressors are, it is easier to identify and implement effective coping strategies, thereby enhancing resilience and preventing burnout.

Professional Development and Leadership

In the context of dentistry, self-knowing is not only concerned with managing emotions but it is also about understanding one's strengths, weaknesses, and areas for growth. Professionals who are self-aware are more open to feedback, more reflective on their practice, and more committed to lifelong learning and continuous professional development. This openness not only benefits their personal development but also enhances the quality of care provided to patients.

This self-awareness is crucial for continuous professional development at all stage of the dental career path. It is also critical for effective leadership within dental teams. The ECR research shows that managers with high self-knowing traits demonstrate strong emotional awareness. They see how their behaviour impacts others (and make changes when they need to). Their body language, tone of voice, and facial expressions are all consistent and easy to read.

Leaders who can accurately assess their strength and development areas are better equipped to inspire and motivate their teams, creating a more positive and productive work environment.

Ethical Practice and Inclusion

Self-knowing also relates to an awareness of one's personal values, biases, and ethical principles. For dental professionals, this holds particular significance in guaranteeing ethical conduct and cultural proficiency. Dental professionals can endeavour to provide equitable care and engage in sensitive interactions with patients from varied backgrounds by engaging in introspection regarding their values and biases. It is important to note that these values and biases will evolve over time and regular reflection is important to acknowledge this. The cultivation of this awareness is crucial in order to effectively tackle health inequities and foster inclusion within the dentistry profession.

Practical Ways to Develop Self-Knowing

Developing self-knowing as a dentist is crucial for personal growth, professional excellence, and the provision of high-quality patient care. Self-awareness, a key component of EI, involves understanding your own emotions, strengths, weaknesses, and values, and recognising their impact on your behaviour and interactions with others. For dentists, who often work in high-pressure environments and deal with anxious patients, cultivating self-awareness can enhance communication skills, decision-making, and patient satisfaction. This section will look at a range of evidence-based strategies to develop this foundational area of EI.

Reflective Practice

Reflective practice is a foundational method for developing self-awareness. It involves critically analysing one's experiences from a personal, patient and staff perspective. The field of Positive Psychology encourages us to reflect on not only the difficult experiences but also those that we have excelled in to identify how we can enhance and develop on the positive learnings. Many studies have highlighted the benefits of reflective practice in dental education, emphasising its role in fostering critical thinking, EI, and self-awareness.

Schön's (1984) model of reflection, which distinguishes between prior-to-action, reflection-in-action and reflection-on-action, offers a framework for this process (see **Table 3.2**).

- *Pre-flective*: This refers to the dentist reflecting before the event, it could be a dentist perhaps writing some notes in a journal before seeing a practical patient that they had difficulty with in a previous encounter. How is the dentist feeling?

Table 3.2 Reflective Approaches

PRACTICE	PRE-FLECTIVE	REFLEXIVE	REFLECTIVE
Reflecting	Prior-to-action	In-action	On-action
Metaphor	Crystal ball	Mirror	Rear-view mirror

Source: Adapted from Schön's Reflective Model (1984).

How might this impact the patient experience? Is there anything they can do to get in a more positive, constructive frame of mind before seeing the patient?
- *Reflexive*: This refers to reflection in real-time when interacting with patients. It is the opportunity to adapt in the moment in response to the situation you find yourself in.
- *Reflective*: This is the most common form of professional reflection and refers to reflecting after the encounter. Considering what went well, what you could do differently next time, key learnings, and so on.

Psychological Safety and Feedback

Feedback from colleagues, mentors, and patients is invaluable for developing self-awareness. Constructive feedback provides insights into areas of strength and opportunities for improvement. It is essential for dentists to create a culture where feedback is regularly sought and given. Psychological Safety should be at the heart of this culture.

Psychological safety is a concept extensively discussed in the field of organisational behaviour, particularly in the work of Amy Edmondson, who has been researching the topic for the last 30 years. According to Edmondson's definition in her seminal 1999 paper 'Psychological Safety and Learning Behaviour in Work Teams,' is defined as "a shared belief held by members of a team that the team is safe for interpersonal risk-taking." It refers to the team climate characterised by interpersonal trust and mutual respect in which people are comfortable being themselves and expressing their opinions without fear of negative consequences to self-image, status, or career.

In environments with high psychological safety, team members feel confident that no one on the team will embarrass or punish anyone else for admitting a mistake, asking a question, or offering feedback. This concept is crucial for fostering an open, inclusive workplace culture where innovation and learning are encouraged, and it has significant implications for teamwork, learning, and performance in organisations.

Emotional Intelligence Training and Profiling

EI training programs specifically designed for healthcare professionals can significantly enhance self-awareness. These programs often include modules on recognising and understanding emotions, managing stress, and empathetic communication. Goleman's EI framework, which identifies self-awareness as a core component, can be particularly useful for dentists. Participating in EI training can help dentists better understand their emotional responses and develop strategies for managing them effectively, leading to improved patient interactions and reduced personal stress.

The RocheMartin ECR is an excellent example of a research-based profile to complete to get metrics on an individual's levels of EI. Each report includes an area to complete a personal development plan based on the results. Ideally this work would be accompanied by a series of coaching sessions to maximise the impact of the work.

Mindfulness and Meditation

Mindfulness and meditation practices are powerful tools for developing self-awareness. These practices involve focusing on the present moment and observing one's thoughts and feelings without judgement. For dentists, who often work in stressful environments, mindfulness can help in recognising stress triggers and managing reactions to them. Studies, such as that of Hülsheger et al. (2013), have shown that mindfulness training can reduce stress, improve focus, and increase emotional regulation, all of which are beneficial for both personal well-being and professional performance.

Professional Development and Continuous Learning

Engaging in continuous professional development and learning is another avenue through which dentists can develop self-awareness. This includes attending workshops, seminars, and conferences, not only on clinical skills but also on communication, leadership, and ethics. Learning new perspectives and skills can challenge existing beliefs and practices, prompting self-reflection and growth. Participation at such events also creates opportunities to grow your network and hence broaden your perspective and outlook. The American Dental Association and other professional bodies often highlight the importance of lifelong learning in maintaining clinical excellence and adapting to the evolving field of dentistry.

Personal Therapy or Coaching

Personal therapy or coaching, especially with a focus on professional roles, can provide a confidential space for dentists to explore their feelings, thoughts, and behaviours. A professional coach or therapist can help identify patterns of behaviour, unconscious biases, and emotional responses that may affect patient care and professional relationships. It is important to distinguish between when coaching is suitable or when therapy is the best option. Generally speaking, therapy is more beneficial when the client needs to deal with emotional trauma or issues from the past blocking them from moving forward in life. Coaching is more related to a future-focused goal setting. This personalised approach of coaching and/or therapy allows for deep self-reflection and the development of targeted strategies to enhance self-awareness and EI.

Social Support Networks

Building and maintaining a supportive social network within and outside the dental profession can contribute to self-awareness. Peer support groups, professional associations, and informal networks provide opportunities for sharing experiences, challenges, and successes. Engaging with peers in discussions about professional issues can offer new insights into one's own practice and highlight common experiences, fostering a sense of community and shared learning.

Professor Rosalind Torres shares interesting research on "What It Takes to Be a Great Leader" in her globally successful TedTalk in 2014. Her studies revealed that three key questions help define successful leadership: Where are you looking to anticipate change? What is the diversity measure of your network? Are you courageous enough to abandon the past? The second question focuses on the importance of having a diverse network of people in your personal and professional life; people from different sociocultural backgrounds, different age groups, different thinking styles, and so on. While it can be more comfortable and convenient to be around people from a similar "tribe" to us, the real growth and learning comes from power of diverse perspectives.

Work–Life Balance

Maintaining a healthy work-life balance is essential for maintaining good levels of self-awareness. Dentists, like other healthcare professionals, can experience burnout due to the challenging nature of their work. Taking time for personal interests, hobbies, and relaxation can help dentists stay connected with their values and interests outside of their professional identity. Building an understanding of where to go to "recharge" is key, this is very personal and often linked to personality styles. For example, people with a preference for extroversion may find they re-energise through activities with other people, for example, playing team sports, socialising. People with a preference for introversion may find this draining and may prefer to do individual activities, for example, cycling or running. This balance is important for emotional well-being and can prevent professional burnout, as suggested by research in fields such as occupational health psychology.

In conclusion, developing self-awareness is a multifaceted process that requires intentional effort and ongoing commitment. For dentists, engaging in reflective practice, seeking feedback, participating in EI training, practising mindfulness, pursuing continuous learning, undergoing personal therapy or coaching, cultivating social support networks, and maintaining a healthy work-life balance are all effective strategies for enhancing self-awareness. By adopting these practices, dentists can improve their ability to understand and manage their emotions, make informed decisions and continue to develop their personal and professional leadership contributing to the well-being of their patients and the communities they serve. For professionals aiming to thrive in their careers, investing in the development of self-awareness is not just beneficial – it is essential. By fostering a deeper understanding of themselves, professionals can unlock their full potential, contributing to their personal growth and the success of their practice.

SELF-KNOWING: DENTAL PRACTITIONER PERSPECTIVE

SALLY HANKS

In dentistry self-knowing is about understanding how and why you respond to specific situations and circumstances in the way you do; how you deal with or manage them (often unconsciously); how that impacts you generally both physically and mentally; and having the self-awareness to develop insight into your own behaviours, reactions, and emotions.

Self-knowing enables the dentist to recognise why certain patterns of behaviour might occur, why and how some professional relationships work better than others and maybe why some don't seem to work at all, and the part each of us plays in these interactions regardless of the words we might choose very carefully.

It is widely recognised and reported that dentistry is a stressful profession. "High levels of self-reported stress, burnout and psychological distress … are a serious concern to the profession" and there are resources for the dental team around well-being and stress management to try to help at a national level (e.g., BDA and NHS).

Like it or not, being a dentist involves constant interactions with colleagues, patients, environments, and within ourselves. Each of us is a human individual with our personal identity, but we also have a professional identity. Perhaps these are closely related, perhaps they are poles apart. Personal identity (who we are) and professional identify (who we and often others think we should be) have been developed in complex ways within each individual, having insight into them will often provide a eureka moment into problems or stresses that seem intransigent, persistent, or recurring.

Within a working day and related to identity is the need for the dentist to inhabit three 'positions' or contexts at once: dentists as individuals as clinicians and as businesspersons. **Figure 3.1** gives an overview of these three positions.

Each of these positions can have contradictory purposes and different decision-making criteria attached to them, leading to stress and/or upset where they are in conflict. Even when a dentist feels they are "doing the right thing" by following best practice guidelines, standards, or protocols, they may be in conflict with themselves unconsciously as the three contexts fight against one another. This idea of having to work within, follow, and apply standard protocols for all patients within the everyday constraints of dental practice is named "articulation work" (Iedema, 2011).

Articulation work can be seen in NHS governance, cross-infection, periodontal treatment protocols, triage levels for seeing emergency patients, and so on.

Where a dentist is trying to run a practice as well as care for patients, often the clinician and businessperson will be in clear conflict. If a dentist is working in a salaried role the

DOI: 10.1201/9781003379829-5

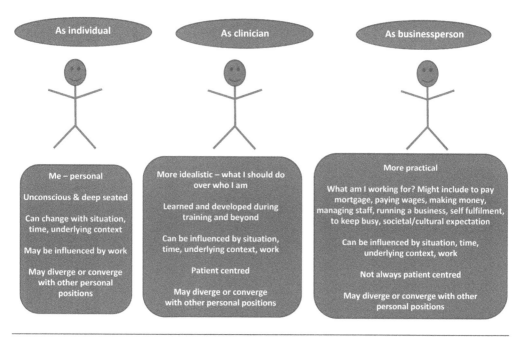

As individual

As clinician

As businessperson

Me – personal	More idealistic – what I should do over who I am	More practical
Unconscious & deep seated	Learned and developed during training and beyond	What am I working for? Might include to pay mortgage, paying wages, making money, managing staff, running a business, self fulfilment, to keep busy, societal/cultural expectation
Can change with situation, time, underlying context	Can be influenced by situation, time, underlying context, work	Can be influenced by situation, time, underlying context, work
May be influenced by work	Patient centred	Not always patient centred
May diverge or converge with other personal positions	May diverge or converge with other personal positions	May diverge or converge with other personal positions

Figure 3.1   The three personal positions or contexts inhabited by dentists within their daily practice.

businessperson element still comes into play, when thinking about constraints made by hierarchy or corporate KPIs, which may go against the individual or clinician perspective.

The interactions between these three positions and the personal and professional identity are reciprocal and ever-changing. They can swing from being in conflict to being fully aligned – when aligned things can feel great. When in conflict things can quickly feel stressful and overwhelming.

Having insight and self-awareness into identity and personal position especially recognising where these might be the basis of emotional responses, non-verbal unconscious communications and behaviours that may cause or lead to stress can in itself start to reduce the stress. It may help identify why it is that that one particular colleague "pushes your buttons," or why your heart sinks when you see that the "difficult patient" is coming in, or why you are drawn toward or avoid specific situations, people, or treatments.

Where there is internal harmony or alignment, there may still be conflict with one or more of the positions or the personal or professional identity and an external source; including a patient, a system such as the NHS or corporate body, an accepted clinical guideline or local community.

Internal and external conflict can lead to tension and emotional stress and influences relationships and decision-making. It can impact patient care as well as practitioner well-being. It may help identify why there is repeated absence, illness, and/or why work impacts so heavily on home life preventing a healthy balance and management of energy for an individual. Self-knowing is the key starting point for developing EI that can make a positive impact on work and leadership.

How to Develop Self-Knowing

Take a breath before responding to a given situation and notice if the intuitive response is actually the one you want to deliver after some cognitive input. Most often the intuitive response comes from the personal position and identity. Thinking and revising a reaction before responding can move it into a more cognitive professional identity space and lead to a more considered behaviour or outcome. It is important however to note that this has been done in order that the associated emotion and effort is not depressed and ignored but acknowledged. Explore your own often deeply held unconscious personal values, beliefs, and assumptions – not to judge but to notice. Learn a skill such as mindfulness or self-hypnosis or seek support from a coach or counsellor if this area of self-development seems too hard or unachievable.

It can be useful to find a trusted colleague as a mentor and be brave enough to wonder and discuss honestly what part you might play in any given situation. Self-knowing plays a fundamental role in the provision of healthcare generally by individual human beings. It can take courage to take an honest "no holds barred" look in the mirror at who we are really; but if we learn to do it, it can help us recognise how and why things are feeling tough, going wrong or why we are not being successful in whatever way we want to be. Professional support in developing self-knowing can be invaluable for enhancing its impact and outcomes.

As a starting point exercise think of a couple of situations that made you feel mildly or moderately uncomfortable or stressed recently. Notice which position has the greatest influence in that situation or more generally. Note which were in conflict and which might be aligned. Think about who you are and who you or others think you should be. It is rare that anyone is in perfect harmony with themselves – but with enhanced self-knowing the negative impact of that can be reduced, and the positives increased.

Examples from Dental Practice

The examples from working as a dentist are ubiquitous and varied and can include attitude to money in general and then how that sits with asking for it for providing healthcare; lack of expertise or aptitude and how that drives either avoidance of a task or development of behaviours and emotions; day to day stressors of managing staff absence or lateness; responding to rude, anxious, fearful, or otherwise "difficult" patients; managing unexpected or unwanted responses from patients, colleagues, or others; running late; having emergency patients squeezed into a busy book; and working within the constraints of a system that one may feel is not fit for purpose; feeling stressed and/or overwhelmed and the coping strategies that are employed to deal with that; impact of work on home life; and having to treat patients or work with colleagues with different political, religious, or social beliefs from one's own.

There follow a couple of specific examples as illustrations.

1. A colleague needs some reasonable adjustments to their role which requires flexible start and finish times.
   - *Individual* – Sympathetic, understanding – or not? Do you welcome change – or not?
   - *Clinician* – Direct or indirect impact on patient bookings, treatment times, surgery support, seeing other people's patients.
   - *Businessperson* – Impact on personal income, practice income, number of patients seen, team/staff relationships, and role allocations.

2. A parent brings in a young child with multiple carious lesions and in pain from abscesses.
   - *Individual* – Are you angry, sad, upset, anxious, bemused, outraged? With the parent? With yourself? With the child?
   - *Clinician* – Thinking about prevention, education for parent and child, treatment, referral. How can this be managed in the best way? How can I do this within the system arrangements (articulation work)? Required skillset and is it available? Do I have it? How to get the child out of pain. A number of appointments are required.
   - *Businessperson* – How will the practice make this work financially? How can I do what I want or need to do within the system/practice/business/contractual arrangements and protocols? I can only have 10 minutes to see this patient – how can I do anything in that time?

References

Babaii A, Mohammadi E, Sadooghiasl A. (2021). The meaning of the empathetic nurse-patient communication: A qualitative study. *J Patient Exp*, *8*, 23743735211056432.

Collin V, Toon M, O'Selmo E, Reynolds L, Whitehead P. (2019). A survey of stress, burnout and well-being in UK dentists. *Br Dent J*, *226*(1), 40–49.

Edmondson A. (1999). Psychological safety and learning behaviour in work teams. *Adm Sci Q*, *44*(2), 350–383.

Hülsheger UR, Alberts HJEM, Feinholdt A, Lang JWB. (2013). Benefits of mindfulness at work: The role of mindfulness in emotion regulation, emotional exhaustion, and job satisfaction. *J Appl Psychol*, *98*(2), 310–325.

Iedema R. (2011). Creating safety by strengthening clinicians' capacity for reflexivity. *BMJ Quality and Safety*, *20*, i83–i86.

Schön DA. (1984). *The Reflective Practitioner: How Professionals Think in Action*, Vol. 5126, Basic Books.

Torres R. (2014). What it takes to be a great leader [internet]. *TedTalks*. https://www.ted.com/talks/roselinde_torres_what_it_takes_to_be_a_great_leader?language=en

4

EQ CRITICAL SKILL II

Self-Control

MARY COLLINS

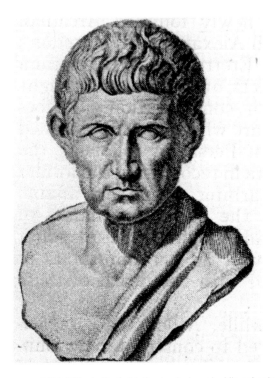

(*Source*: https://www.gettyimages.co.uk/detail/illustration/aristotle-classical-greek-philosopher-he-is-royalty-free-illustration/1408233961?adppopup=true)

Introduction

The ancient Greek philosopher, Aristotle, describes the importance of self-control and moderation in his writings. One of his notable quotes on the control of emotions is:

> I count him braver who overcomes his desires than him who conquers his enemies; for the hardest victory is over self.

This quote highlights the significance of mastering one's emotions and desires as a form of bravery and strength. He considered self-control and the ability to manage one's impulses as a greater victory than defeating external adversaries, emphasising the importance of inner discipline and emotional regulation.

DOI: 10.1201/9781003379829-6

This chapter will explore the following elements of self-control as a critical skill for dentists at all career stages:

- A definition of self-control
- Importance of this area in dentistry across all career stages
- Practical ways to develop self-control
- Dental practitioner perspective

Definition of Self-Control

Self-control is a critical competency of emotional intelligence that plays a pivotal role in personal and professional development. The competency is described in the Emotional Capital Report as managing emotions well and restraining actions until there is time to think rationally. This prevents their behaviour from being governed by moods and emotions. Self-control is about demonstrating calmness and level-headedness under pressure.

It is the ability to manage disruptive emotions and impulses effectively, to think before acting, and to maintain a focus on goals despite setbacks and challenges. It encompasses not merely the restraint of negative emotions but also the channelling of emotions towards constructive outcomes.

At its core, self-control is about the ability to regulate one's emotional responses, it is about "responding not reacting." This involves recognising when an emotion or impulse is likely to lead to undesirable outcomes and taking steps to adjust that response in favour of a more desirable or productive outcome. It is the capacity to pause and choose how to act, rather than being swept away by immediate reactions. This competency is crucial in high-pressure environments where decisions must be made in a considered way to avoid negative consequences.

Self-control is a critical element of emotional intelligence because it directly impacts an individual's ability to navigate complex social environments, make rational decisions, and achieve long-term goals. It supports other aspects of emotional intelligence, such as self-awareness, by requiring an individual to manage their emotional states. It also enhances social skills by enabling individuals to respond to interpersonal challenges with patience and empathy, rather than reactive negative emotions.

Self-control plays a critical role in shaping workplace dynamics, influencing everything from leadership behaviours, individual performance to team cohesion. Its presence or absence can significantly impact the professional environment, affecting decision-making, interpersonal relationships, and overall productivity. Understanding the behaviours associated with high and low self-control can provide insights into personal development needs and strategies for improving workplace interactions.

Table 4.1 shares behaviours seen in the workplace when Self-Control is high and also when it is lacking.

Table 4.1   Self-Control: Behaviours of High and Low Levels in the Workplace

HIGH SELF-CONTROL BEHAVIOURS AT WORK	LOW SELF-CONTROL BEHAVIOURS AT WORK
When someone possesses a high level of self-control, we see the following characteristics in their behaviour and interactions:	When someone possesses a low level of self-control, we see the following characteristics in their behaviour and interactions:
1. *Measured responses to stress*: People with high self-control can manage stress effectively, responding to challenging situations with calmness and composure. Instead of reacting impulsively to stress triggers, they take a step back, assess the situation, and choose the best course of action.	1. *Impulsiveness*: Low self-control often manifests as impulsive behaviour, with individuals reacting rashly to situations without considering the consequences. This impulsivity can lead to poor decision-making, mistakes, and interpersonal conflict.
2. *Constructive conflict resolution*: High self-control facilitates positive conflict resolution. Individuals are more likely to listen actively, consider different perspectives, and seek solutions that benefit all stakeholders involved.	2. *Difficulty handling stress*: Professionals who have difficulty regulating emotions may become easily overwhelmed by stress. This can manifest as anxiety, frustration, or even withdrawal, impacting their performance and well-being.
3. *Consistent performance*: Self-control is linked to the ability to resist distractions and stay focused on tasks. Employees with this trait can set priorities, manage their time efficiently, and maintain high levels of productivity, even when faced with potential disruptions.	3. *Poor time management*: A lack of self-control can make it difficult for individuals to avoid distractions and stay on task. This often results in procrastination, missed deadlines, and inconsistent work quality.
4. *Positive workplace relationships*: High self-control contributes to patience, empathy, and effective communication in relation to interpersonal interactions. Such individuals are skilled at navigating social dynamics, building trust, and fostering positive relationships.	4. *Difficult interpersonal relationships*: Low self-control can strain workplace relationships. Impatience, lack of empathy, and ineffective communication can lead to misunderstandings and conflicts, impacting trust and cooperation among team members.
5. *Ethical standards*: Self-control is critical for maintaining professional integrity. It underpins the ability to uphold ethical standards, resist temptations that could lead to unethical behaviour, and make principled decisions.	5. *Compromised ethics*: In extreme cases, low self-control can result in unethical behaviour or unprofessional conduct. The inability to resist temptations or manage impulses can have serious repercussions for both the individual and the organisation.

High Self-Control in the Workplace

When self-control is high among professionals in the workplace, several positive behaviours and outcomes become evident:

1. *Measured responses to stress*: People with high self-control can manage stress effectively, responding to challenging situations with calmness and composure. Instead of reacting impulsively to stress triggers, they take a step back, assess the situation, and choose the best course of action.

2. *Constructive conflict resolution*: High self-control facilitates positive conflict resolution. Individuals are more likely to listen actively, consider different perspectives, and seek solutions that benefit all stakeholders involved.

3. *Consistent performance*: Self-control is linked to the ability to resist distractions and stay focused on tasks. Employees with this trait can set priorities, manage their time efficiently, and maintain high levels of productivity, even when faced with potential disruptions.

4. *Positive workplace relationships*: High self-control contributes to patience, empathy, and effective communication in relation to interpersonal interactions. Such individuals are skilled at navigating social dynamics, building trust, and fostering positive relationships.

5. *Ethical standards*: Self-control is critical for maintaining professional integrity. It underpins the ability to uphold ethical standards, resist temptations that could lead to unethical behaviour, and make principled decisions.

Low Self-Control in the Workplace

When self-control is low, a range of negative behaviours and outcomes can be seen in the workplace:

1. *Impulsiveness*: Low self-control often manifests as impulsive behaviour, with individuals reacting rashly to situations without considering the consequences. This impulsivity can lead to poor decision-making, mistakes, and interpersonal conflict.

2. *Difficulty handling stress*: Professionals who have difficulty regulating emotions may become easily overwhelmed by stress. This can manifest as anxiety, frustration, or even withdrawal, impacting their performance and well-being.

3. *Poor time management*: A lack of self-control can make it difficult for individuals to avoid distractions and stay on task. This often results in procrastination, missed deadlines, and inconsistent work quality.

4. *Difficult interpersonal relationships*: Low self-control can strain workplace relationships. Impatience, lack of empathy, and ineffective communication can lead to misunderstandings and conflicts, impacting trust and cooperation among team members.

5. *Compromised ethics*: In extreme cases, low self-control can result in unethical behaviour or unprofessional conduct. The inability to resist temptations or manage impulses can have serious repercussions for both the individual and the organisation.

Importance of Self-Control in Dentistry

Emotional self-control, a key area of emotional intelligence, plays an important role in the dental profession. The ability to manage and regulate one's emotions, especially in high-stress situations, not only enhances personal well-being but also significantly impacts professional relationships, patient care, and overall career success. It is imperative that dentists cultivate emotional self-control from their time as students until they reach retirement in order to confront the rigours and expectations of the field while maintaining their professionalism and resilience.

Dental Students

Dental education is not just about acquiring technical expertise; it's also a critical period for developing the emotional competencies necessary for effective practice. Emotional self-control for dental students involves managing the stress of rigorous academic and clinical training while maintaining a positive and growth-oriented mindset.

Students must learn to work collaboratively with peers, instructors, and patients. Emotional self-control facilitates constructive feedback, teamwork, and having a positive experience with the first stages of patient interaction.

Early Career Dentists

The transition from student to practising dentist can be a challenging time dealing with situations including the stress of establishing oneself in the profession, managing a practice, and dealing with patients. Emotional self-control allows new dentists to deal with these challenges without being overwhelmed, making more reasoned decisions and building strong patient rapport.

Developing emotional self-control early in one's career develops resilience, a critical quality for long-term career satisfaction and success. It enables dentists to face setbacks and criticism constructively, seeing them as opportunities for growth rather than threats.

Mid-Career Dentists

As dentists progress in their careers, many take on leadership roles, either by running their own practices or leading teams within larger organisations. Emotional self-control is crucial for effective leadership, allowing dentists to inspire and motivate their staff, manage conflicts, and maintain a positive practice environment.

Mid-career professionals often face the challenge of balancing professional responsibilities with personal and family commitments. Emotional self-control helps in managing these competing demands, preventing burnout, and maintaining a healthy work–life balance.

Late Career and Retirement

In the later stages of their careers, dentists often focus on mentoring younger professionals and leaving a legacy. Emotional self-control enhances their ability to provide thoughtful, considered guidance, navigate the challenges of mentorship, and handle the emotional aspects of approaching retirement.

Retirement is a significant life transition that can evoke a wide range of emotions. For retiring dentists, emotional self-control facilitates this transition, allowing them to find fulfilment in retirement and adapt to their new life stage. They can adjust to the new life phase in a calm, considered way by dealing with the range of emotions at this time in a positive, constructive way.

Strategies to Develop Emotional Self-Control

Developing self-control is essential for dentists who aim to excel in all aspects of their profession. Good self-control is the cornerstone of maintaining positive relationships with patients and staff and maintaining personal well-being. Self-control, as part of the emotional intelligence framework, involves managing one's emotions and impulses to respond to various situations in a considered and effective manner. For dentists, who often work in high-stress environments and deal with anxious patients, mastering self-control can significantly impact the quality of care provided and the overall workplace atmosphere.

Recognising the signs of low self-control is the first step toward improvement. Developing this crucial skill requires a conscious effort to understand and manage emotions, set and pursue considered goals, and practice restraint in the face of provocations or stress triggers. Below are a range of practical suggestions to developing self-control at a personal level, with patients, and among staff.

Personal Level

The journey to developing self-control involves various strategies that focus on both the mind and body, that when mastered, significantly enhance one's quality of life. Below are suggestions on how to cultivate self-control on a personal level:

- **Practice Mindfulness and Meditation**
  - *Daily practice*: Begin your day with a simple daily routine, start by dedicating 5–10 minutes and build up over time if this approach works for you. Apps can be helpful to provide a guided practice, for example, Headspace and Calm Apps.
  - *Integration into daily life*: Beyond starting your day with meditation, consider integrating mindfulness into routine activities. This can include mindful eating, where you pay full attention to the taste and texture of your food, or mindful walking, where you focus on the sensation of your feet touching the ground. These practices help embed mindfulness throughout your day, not just in isolated moments.
  - *Community support*: Joining a mindfulness group or community can provide additional motivation and insight. Sharing experiences and tips with others can deepen your practice and offer new perspectives on managing stress and emotions.
  - *Impact*: A consistent mindfulness practice enhances awareness of your emotional states and triggers, improving your ability to manage stress.

It has also been shown to physically alter regions of the brain associated with memory, empathy, and stress regulation. Over time, this can lead to significant improvements in emotional well-being, resilience, and overall mental health (Hölzel et al., 2011).

- **Set Personal Goals**
  - *How*: Develop SMART (specific, measurable, achievable, realistic, time-bound) goals for your personal and professional life. Regularly review and adjust these goals as necessary.
  - *Visualisation*: In addition to setting SMART goals, incorporate visualisation techniques. Imagine not just achieving your goals but also the steps you will take to get there. Neuroscience research shows how this process can increase motivation and clarify the path forward.
  - *Public commitment*: Sharing your goals with others can significantly increase your accountability. Whether it's with a friend, family member, or on social media, making your goals public can provide an extra layer of motivation.
  - *Impact*: Positive psychology research informs us that having a sense of accomplishment is key to leading a fulfilled life. Having clear, realistic goals helps maintain focus and motivation. Regular review of progress against these goals reduces the likelihood of being swayed by distractions or emotional triggers.
  - *Goal-setting*, when done correctly, not only provides direction but also serves as a potent source of motivation. It aligns your focus with your values and aspirations, making daily tasks more meaningful and reducing procrastination (Locke and Latham, 2002).

- **Regular Physical Activity**
  - *How*: Incorporate physical exercise into your daily routine, find an activity that suits your personality and one that you enjoy to maximise the likelihood to committing to the exercise practice.
  - *Variety in exercise*: To stop your exercise routine from being mundane, introduce variety. Mixing different types of physical activities can prevent boredom and promote a more comprehensive approach to fitness. This can include a combination of cardiovascular exercises, strength training, flexibility exercises, and balance training.
  - *Track progress*: Use apps or a journal to track your exercise progress. Seeing improvements over time can be a significant motivational booster and help in setting more challenging goals.
  - *Impact*: Exercise is not only excellent for physical help but is a powerful stress reliever and mood booster. This supports emotional regulation and stress reduction and builds "a buffer" of resilience for meeting the challenges of work and life. Regular physical activity can improve sleep quality, increase self-esteem, and reduce symptoms of mental health conditions like depression and anxiety (Chekroud et al., 2018).

- **Seek Constructive Feedback**
  - *How*: Regularly ask for feedback from peers, mentors, or team members on your handling of stressful situations and emotional responses. The best time to seek feedback is close to the time of the stressful event but allow enough space after so that you are in a position to receive the feedback in a calm, composed way. A more formal, structured approach is through a 360-feedback process, where you receive anonymous feedback from a range of sources (typically around 10–14 people including line managers, peers, direct reports, and others). 360 feedback is most successful if supported with an executive coach to work with the individual to build a development plan based on the feedback.
  - *Reflection and action*: After receiving feedback, take time to reflect on it critically and develop an action plan for improvement. This reflection process turns feedback into a constructive tool for personal development.
  - *Creating a feedback culture*: Encourage a culture of continuous feedback within your personal and professional circles. This could mean regularly asking for feedback and also offering constructive feedback to others, fostering a mutual growth environment.
  - *Impact*: Constructive feedback is invaluable for personal development. It raises self-awareness by providing insights into behaviour and areas for improvement, fostering personal growth. Builds psychological trust within the team but creating a culture when feedback is given and received with ease and respect. It highlights blind spots in our behaviour and thinking patterns, offering a clear direction for growth and improvement.

- **Develop Coping Strategies**
  - *Education on stress management*: Educate yourself on the physiological and psychological aspects of stress. Understanding stress's effects on your body and mind can demystify experiences of stress and empower you with the knowledge to combat it effectively.

    Identify stressors in your practice and personal life. Understand that coping strategies should be personalised. What works for one person may not work for another. Experiment with different techniques, such as yoga, journaling, or hobbies that relax and recharge you, to find what best helps you manage stress.

    This can be supported by working with a coach, mentor or a therapist for deeper emotion work.
  - *Impact*: Effective stress management not only improves your immediate mental and physical well-being but also has long-term health benefits. It can decrease the risk of chronic diseases associated with stress, such as hypertension, heart disease, and diabetes.

By adopting these strategies, individuals can significantly enhance their ability to exercise self-control in various aspects of their life, leading to a more balanced, successful, and fulfilling existence. Each approach, from mindfulness to setting personal goals, plays a crucial role in building a foundation for strong self-control.

With Patients

Developing self-control in patient interactions is essential for dentists to maintain a professional and supportive dental practice environment. Below are some suggestions for dentists to further enhance their ability to manage themselves effectively in various patient scenarios:

- **Practice Empathetic Listening**
  - *Active listening techniques*: Focus entirely on the patient while they speak, avoiding distractions and interrupting. Nod and provide affirmative sounds or words to show you are engaged.
  - *Reflect and validate*: After the patient finishes speaking, reflect back what you heard and validate their feelings. This could be as simple as "It sounds like you're really worried about this procedure, and that's completely understandable."
  - *Impact*: Empathetic listening has been linked to better patient outcomes and higher satisfaction levels (Berry, 2001). It establishes trust and builds rapport with patients making it easier to manage their anxiety and increases compliance with treatment plans.

Such practices can also reduce the dentist's own stress levels, as understanding patient concerns can lead to more effective communication and treatment planning.

- **Communicate Clearly and Calmly**
  - *How*: Use simple, jargon-free language to explain diagnoses, procedures, and expectations. Remain calm and composed, even in the face of patient anxiety or dissatisfaction.
  - *Educational materials*: Share visuals or models to help explain complex procedures. This can aid in ensuring the patient understands what to expect.
  - *Feedback loop*: After explaining, ask patients to summarise their understanding. This checks for comprehension and allows you to clarify as needed.
  - *Impact*: Clear communication is associated with improved patient outcomes and reduced malpractice claims. When patients understand their treatment, they are less anxious and more cooperative (Levinson et al., 2010).

Maintaining calm, especially in challenging interactions, models emotional regulation for patients, potentially de-escalating tense situations and promoting a more positive clinical environment and smooth running of the practice.

- **Set Boundaries**
  - *How*: Clearly communicate practice policies, appointment schedules, and treatment protocols to patients. Be firm yet empathetic in enforcing these boundaries.
  - *Consistent policies*: Ensure that all staff members are trained on practice policies and can communicate them clearly and consistently to patients.
  - *Advance communication*: Use appointment reminders to reiterate policies on cancellations or late arrivals. This proactive communication can help manage expectations. Over-communication is preferable to under-communication!
  - *Impact*: Setting and maintaining boundaries is crucial for time management and practice efficiency. It helps in managing patient flow and ensuring that each patient receives the attention they need.

Clear boundaries also contribute to a better work-life balance for dentists by reducing after-hours calls and stress, contributing to overall job satisfaction, and reducing burnout.

Incorporating these strategies into daily practice allows dentists to foster a positive, respectful, and empathetic relationship with their patients. This not only enhances patient care but also supports dentists in managing their emotional and professional responses more effectively, leading to a more rewarding practice environment.

With Staff

Developing self-control within the context of a dental practice extends beyond patient interactions; it is critical in managing relationships with staff. Here is how dentists can lead their teams effectively by modelling self-control and fostering a supportive work environment:

- **Lead by Example**
  - *Model emotional regulation*: Actively demonstrate how to handle stress and unexpected issues calmly and professionally. Share and practice stress management techniques, like mindfulness or short meditative breaks, during the workday.
    - This could simply include taking a moment to breathe before responding to a challenging situation.
  - *Impact*: By leading through example, dentists set the tone for the entire office. Research shows that leaders' emotional regulation and coping strategies significantly influence the workplace atmosphere and employee well-being (Goleman, 1998).
    - This leadership approach encourages a culture where staff feel motivated to model these positive behaviours, leading to a more resilient and adaptive team.

- **Encourage Open Communication**
  - *How*: Create a psychologically safe environment where staff feel comfortable voicing concerns, suggestions, and feedback without fear of retribution.
  - *Regular feedback sessions*: Implement regular one-on-one feedback sessions with staff, offering a safe space for open dialogue.
  - *Team-building activities*: Organise team-building activities supported by experts, for example, workplace psychologists, that emphasise communication and trust, reinforcing the importance of a supportive team environment.
  - *Impact*: Open communication fosters a sense of belonging and teamwork, making it easier to navigate conflicts and challenges, thus maintaining a smoother operational flow within the practice.
    - A psychologically safe workplace encourages staff to share ideas, concerns, and feedback, which is crucial for innovation and solving complex problems (Edmondson, 1999).

- **Provide Support and Resources**
  - *How*: Offer training and supports (e.g., employee assistance programme) for stress management. Recognise and address signs of burnout among staff. Implement wellness programmes that include stress management workshops and access to mental health resources.
  - *Recognition programmes*: Develop recognition programmes to celebrate staff achievements and milestones, promoting a positive and supportive work environment.
  - *Impact*: Offering resources for personal and professional development promotes staff well-being and job satisfaction, which are directly linked to patient satisfaction and practice success.

Acknowledging and addressing signs of burnout not only helps in retaining staff but also ensures that the quality of patient care is not compromised due to staff fatigue or disengagement.

- **Conduct Regular Team Meetings**
  - *How*: Schedule frequent meetings to talk about patient care, practice management, and any issues. Use these meetings as an opportunity to practice and reinforce emotional regulation strategies.
  - *Structured agendas*: Ensure meetings have a clear, structured agenda that allows time for discussing patient care, practice updates, and staff concerns in a structured manner.
  - *Emotional regulation focus*: Incorporate a segment in meetings dedicated to discussing and practising emotional regulation strategies, reinforcing their importance in the workplace. For example, this could be simply starting each meeting with a "mindful moment" of breathing to set the tone for a calm, composed, efficient meeting.

- *Impact*: Regular team meetings ensure that all staff members are aligned with the practice's goals and operational standards, fostering a sense of unity and purpose (Lencioni, 2002).

These gatherings also serve as a platform for collective problem-solving and innovation, promoting a cooperative and harmonious work environment by making sure everyone is aligned and working towards shared objectives.

By focusing on these areas, dentists can lead their teams more effectively, creating a work environment that not only fosters professional growth and high-quality patient care but also enhances the overall well-being and satisfaction of the staff.

Conclusion

Emotional self-control is a cornerstone of emotional intelligence that significantly influences a dentist's ability to manage stress, build positive relationships, and achieve professional success. Developing this skill requires ongoing effort and reflection but offers profound benefits across the dental career lifespan.

In a world that often values immediate gratification and reactive responses, self-control remains a key differentiator for individuals seeking to lead a balanced, successful, and fulfilling life.

Developing self-control is a continuous journey that requires dedication and practice. By focusing on personal growth, fostering positive patient interactions, and leading a supportive team environment, dentists can significantly enhance their professional practice and personal life. Implementing the practical approaches outlined above can lead to improved emotional regulation, better decision-making, and stronger relationships with both patients and staff, ultimately contributing to a successful and rewarding dental career.

SELF-CONTROL: DENTAL PRACTITIONER PERSPECTIVE

SALLY HANKS

What Is Self-Control

Patients expect their healthcare providers to know what they are doing and then to do it, in the best way for them as a patient. It is where trust emanates from. Trust is essential for effective care to be provided (Goold, 2002).

Self-control is about managing one's own emotions and reactions, while dealing with others' emotions and behaviours at the same time. It involves discipline and competence, and a level of self-confidence to enable appropriate control to be maintained in a given situation.

Patients are a unique group of people because they are often vulnerable and in need of the expertise of the healthcare provider, creating a power imbalance in the relationship. They may lack understanding and knowledge of the situation they are in. They are out of control of the situation, and the self-control of the clinician is fundamental to enable an effective interaction to take place so that the patient feels some sense of control being returned to them.

Self-control is the ability to think rationally and cognitively and let that guide the situation in place of emotional thinking and reactions. Being guided by such rational, cognitive thoughts which are not necessarily congruent with the emotions being felt is called emotional labour and immaterial labour.

Numerous authors explain the issue of emotional labour where individuals are required to manage their own emotions (emotional regulation) while concurrently portraying a specific, non-emotional reaction to their clients as part of their job (Haver et al., 2013; Held and McKimm, 2011; Nicolson et al., 2011). Emotional labour involves successful self-regulation and explicit self-awareness, alongside being able to manage a patient's emotions and the potential conflict a situation may provoke. This whole is described as immaterial labour (Iedema et al., 2006) where a practitioner may have to spontaneously discuss, redesign, or evaluate their situated interactions in face-to-face communications, while also dealing with others' (e.g., patients, colleagues, system representatives) views, feelings, or emotions.

Self-control requires the discipline to take a step back and not react, alongside the ability to think rationally and exude an air of calmness at the same time.

Why Is Self-Control Important in Dentistry?

As a dentist it is common to hear the statement "I hate dentists" as the patient walks into a surgery. Other common reports relate to how much money dentists are perceived to have, how they enjoy inflicting pain and putting knees on chests to get teeth

DOI: 10.1201/9781003379829-7

out, and how if they were not so greedy there would be more affordable care for everyone. These attitudes are often portrayed in the media as well as by individuals and so are exacerbated and promulgated as fact. Patients show us a range of emotions as they undergo care at our hands including being anxious, scared, panicking, angry, upset, and confused. They can demonstrate a range of behaviours and responses that make caregiving more difficult, time-consuming, and frustrating, including being reluctant, stubborn, argumentative, not listening, not believing, being rude, personal or depersonalising, and responding unpredictably.

In the face of all this the dentist has to maintain an air of calmness, intelligent kindness, compassion, and competence. This has to be done in an authentic way to ensure negative or highly charged situations are not escalated and to maintain trust that they know what they are doing and are doing it in the best interests of their patient.

Most often in a dental practice a patient is undergoing treatment that they do not necessarily want, and that is not very pleasant to undergo. Then they have to pay their hard-earned money for it.

Additionally, in the practice there are staff to work with and manage, systems that can create restraints and frustration, interruptions or changes to the day's planned proceedings, personal needs or wants that have to be ignored/saved for later, personal emotions and life events that impact mood and well-being (including illness, bereavement, family arguments, worry about loved ones), financial obligations, complaints – the list could go on and on.

Dentists are human beings. Having the discipline, calmness and ability to think rationally is a difficult skill. It is required alongside high levels of self-knowing in order to acknowledge the skill and work being done. Without the reflection on the interaction between these two areas, it would be easy to develop severe stress, burnout, and/or compassion fatigue.

Burnout will often lead to depression, and stress increases the risk of developing mental health conditions such as depression, alcoholism, sleeplessness, and drug addiction (Denton et al., 2008). The highest reported consequence of stress and also the one reported to impact most on family life outside of work is nervousness (Myers and Myers, 2004) with a recent report suggesting that, "the high levels of self-reported stress, burnout & psychological distress … are a serious concern to the profession" (Collin et al., 2019).

Dentists leave the profession early not only from back problems, but stress-related illness, and there is the often-reported risk of suicide. While studies and articles debate whether or not dentists are at higher risk than other professions and the general public of suicide, the risk itself cannot be ignored. The insight and self-awareness into the levels of self-control required can help mitigate the risk (Bradley, 2020).

One of the biggest reported stressors in dental practice is being complained about and having to undergo a formal investigation or Fitness to Practise process by the regulator. These investigations often take many months or years to complete and can create huge amounts of upset and worry. Being able to continue to work – sometimes with the patient or colleague who has raised the complaint or concern against you – is often required and the levels of self-control required for such situations can feel almost superhuman. Development activities and sufficient decompensation will be needed if a dentist finds themselves in such a situation.

How to Develop Self-Control

As with many of the emotional intelligence competencies required for effective practice, a bit of space for self-reflection and metacognition on practice can start the development of self-control. Looking at situations from the day – when things went well or not – and noticing the behaviours and the emotions involved consciously, rather than allowing the day to go by and the work to all be done intuitively or unconsciously. Taking a breath or a moment to be still, working with a coach, counsellor or mentor, and reading about the skills of self-control can also help.

It can be useful to create strategies that can be used in the moment. In a dental surgery, it may not be easy to remove the dentist from the situation to enable them to take a break, but perhaps taking a moment to wash hands or check something on the computer. Most of the time in a dental setting the patient is lying or sitting in the chair and to look at the computer or stand up and wash hands means turning away from the patient. Both these approaches give the dentist a short respite from being directly in the patient's gaze, and it can bring a few moments in which to reset. Having opportunities for debriefing can be useful – formally or informally – this is often best done within the practice or with a trusted colleague/professional because of the importance of maintaining patient confidentiality.

In addition to having strategies to develop self-control and insight into when and how it is manifested in daily practice, sufficient decompensation activities are useful in general. This is as much about managing energy as it is time – it is often not under the dentist's control how much time is spent in the surgery at work – there will be multiple burdens and obligations that impact that – and so it is about managing energy. Decompensation activities can range from running marathons and going to the gym for hours, to a daily 15-minute mental, emotional, or spiritual practice including yoga, mindfulness, and meditation as examples. Each dentist's need for intuitive and conscious levels of self-control will vary depending on their individual context, and so calming and restoring activities may also need to differ. Each individual should determine what works for them, and then make time to do it. The discipline of making time for that will, in itself, support the development of self-control, and so this becomes a virtuous cycle.

Examples from Dental Practice

The previous paragraphs have highlighted a plethora of nonspecific times and situations during the working day of a dental practice where self-control is vital. Below are examples of specific situations but there are almost an infinite array of examples a dentist will have to manage during their working life.

Your nurse has complained about you to the practice manager for bullying. There is to be an internal investigation and while that is ongoing you are having to continue to work with the same nurse.

Your colleague is off sick and this is the fourth day off they have taken in as many weeks. You are having to cover their patients as well as your own.

The receptionist has "squeezed in" an emergency patient at the end of your working day. It is not a name you recognise but when you review the notes, you realise that it is a patient that you find very difficult to treat because of their high levels of anxiety. You have previously given in-depth advice about their condition and how they can manage it at home – you perceive that they are not heeding your advice and doing what they have always done instead.

You get home from work after a day that you have found more tiring than usual. You feel short-tempered and in need of a bit of quiet and some space. You are asked a question, snap a reply, and get into an argument almost as soon as you have got in. And you have been admonished for being later than you said you would be.

Your patient says that they need to take sips of water throughout treatment because having their mouth open makes them cough.

You are performing an extraction and hear a loud cracking noise. The patient is visibly upset and starts to panic.

References

Berry P. (2001) From detached concern to empathy: Humanizing medical practice. *BMJ*, 323 (7325): 1373.

Bradley N. (2020). Suicide and dentistry: An unwanted link. *BDJ in Pract*, 33 (5): 20–21.

Collin V, Toon M, O'Selmo E, Reynolds L, Whitehead P. (2019) A survey of stress, burnout and well-being in UK dentists. *Br Dent J*, 226 (1): 40–49.

Chekroud SR, Gueorguieva R, Zheutlin AB, Paulus M, Krumholz HM, Krystal JH, Chekroud AM. (2018) Association between physical exercise and mental health in 1–2 million individuals in the USA between 2011 and 2015: A cross-sectional study. *Lancet Psychiatry*, 5 (9): 739–746.

Denton DA, Newton JT, Bower EJ. (2008) Occupational burnout and work engagement: A national survey of dentists in the United Kingdom. *Br Dent J*, 20 (7): E13.

Edmondson A. (1999) Psychological safety and learning behaviour in work teams. *Administrative Science Q*, 44 (2): 350–383.

Goleman D. (1998). The emotional intelligence of leaders. *Leader to Leader*, 10 (5): 20–26.

Goold SD. (2002) Trust, distrust and trustworthiness. *J Gen Intern Med*, 17 (1): 79–81.

Haver A, Akerjordet K, Furunes T. (2013). Emotion regulation and its implications for leadership: An integrative review and future research agenda. *J Leadersh Org Stud*, 20 (5): 287–303.

Held S, McKimm J. (2011) Emotional intelligence, emotional labour and affective leadership, in Preedy M, Bennett N, Wise C, eds. Educational Leadership: Context, Strategy and Collaboration. Open University/Sage: 52–64.

Hölzel BK, Carmody J, Vangel M, Congleton C, Yerramsetti SM, Gard T, Lazar SW. (2011) Mindfulness practice leads to increases in regional brain gray matter density. *Psychiatry Res*, 191 (1): 36–43.

Iedema R, Long D, Forsyth R, Lee BB. (2006) Visibilizing clinical work: Video ethnography in the contemporary hospital. *Health Sociol Rev*, 15: 156–168.

Lencioni Patrick. (2002). *The Five Dysfunctions of a Team*. New York, NY: Jossey-Bass.

Levinson W, Lesser CS, Epstein RM. (2010) Developing physician communication skills for patient-centered care. *Health Aff*, 29 (7): 1310–1318.

Locke EA, Latham GP. (2002). Building a practically useful theory of goal setting and task motivation: A 35-year odyssey. *American Psychologist*, 57 (9): 705–717.

Myers HL, Myers LB. (2004). 'It's difficult being a dentist': Stress and health in the general dental practitioner. *Br Dent J*, 197 (5): 89–93.

Nicolson P, Rowland E, Lokman P, Fox R, Gabriel Y, Heffernan K, Howorth C, Ilan-Clarke Y, Smith G. (2011) Leadership and Better Patient Care: Managing in the NHS. Final Report [internet]. NIHR Service Delivery and Organisation Programme. Available at https://www.netscc.ac.uk/hsdr/files/project/SDO_FR_08-1601-137_V01.pdf (accessed December 2016).

EQ CRITICAL SKILL III

Empathy

MARY COLLINS

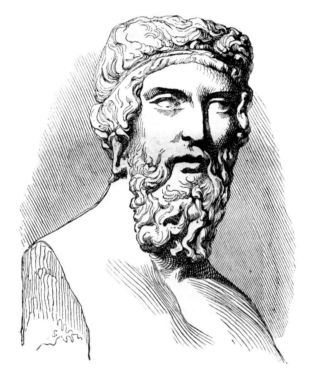

Introduction

Plato, the ancient Greek philosopher, offered insights into human nature and ethics that have been interpreted to encompass the concept of empathy. One quote that reflects this is: "Be kind, for everyone you meet is fighting a hard battle."

This quote reminds us that everyone has their own struggles and challenges, many of which are not immediately visible. It encourages us to approach all interactions with kindness and understanding, recognising the shared human experience of overcoming difficulties.

DOI: 10.1201/9781003379829-8

This chapter will focus on the following topics in relation to the core area of empathy in dentistry:

- Definition of empathy
- Why is empathy important at all stages of the dental career journey?
- Empathy and litigation
- Practical strategies to develop empathy
- Dental practitioner perspective

Definition of Empathy

Empathy, as defined within the framework of the RocheMartin Emotional Capital Report, is about being adept at understanding and taking into account other people's thoughts and feelings. Using attentive listening to build rapport, demonstrate curiosity about others, and establish strong emotional connections with others by focusing on and validating their feelings.

Empathy is a foundational element of emotional intelligence that refers to the capacity to understand and share the feelings of another. This competency goes beyond mere sympathy to entail a deeper, more intuitive grasp of the perspectives and emotional states of others. In the context of the workplace, especially within healthcare settings, empathy manifests through various behaviours and significantly impacts interactions, decision-making, and the overall environment (**Table 5.1**).

High Empathy in the Workplace

When empathy levels are high among healthcare professionals and staff, several positive behaviours become evident:

1. *Active listening*: Individuals demonstrate an authentic interest in understanding others' points of view, encouraging open and honest communication. They pay close attention not just to the words being said but also to the non-verbal cues, such as tone of voice and body language.
2. *Understanding and compassion*: Employees show a genuine concern for the feelings and well-being of colleagues and patients. This is reflected in their approach to care, where they consider the patient's emotional and psychological needs alongside their physical health needs.
3. *Constructive feedback*: Empathetic individuals provide feedback in a way that is sensitive to the recipient's feelings. They frame their observations and suggestions in a supportive manner, aimed at fostering growth rather than causing distress.
4. *Conflict resolution*: High empathy contributes to more effective conflict resolution strategies. Understanding the emotional underpinnings of conflicts allows for resolutions that address the concerns of all parties involved.

Table 5.1   Empathy: Behaviours of High and Low Levels in the Workplace

HIGH-EMPATHY BEHAVIOURS AT WORK	LOW-EMPATHY BEHAVIOURS AT WORK
When someone possesses a high level of empathy, we see the following characteristics in their behaviour and interactions:	When someone possesses a low level of empathy, we see the following characteristics in their behaviour and interactions:
1. *Active listening*: Individuals demonstrate an authentic interest in understanding others' points of view, encouraging open-and-honest communication. They pay close attention not just to the words being said but also to the non-verbal cues, such as tone of voice and body language. 2. *Understanding and compassion*: Employees show a genuine concern for the feelings and well-being of colleagues and patients. This is reflected in their approach to care, where they consider the patient's emotional and psychological needs alongside their physical health needs. 3. *Constructive feedback*: Empathetic individuals provide feedback in a way that is sensitive to the recipient's feelings. They frame their observations and suggestions in a supportive manner, aimed at fostering growth rather than causing distress. 4. *Conflict resolution*: High empathy contributes to more effective conflict resolution strategies. Understanding the emotional underpinnings of conflicts allows for resolutions that address the concerns of all parties involved. 5. *Positive work environment*: An empathetic workplace fosters a culture of mutual respect, understanding, and collaboration. This leads to higher job satisfaction, employee retention, and a supportive atmosphere.	1. *Miscommunication*: A lack of empathy often leads to misunderstandings and misinterpretations, as individuals may not fully consider the perspectives or emotional states of their colleagues or patients. 2. *Reduced patient satisfaction*: In healthcare settings, low empathy can result in patient care that feels impersonal, rushed, or uncaring. This can lead to decreased patient satisfaction and trust in healthcare providers. 3. *Increased conflict*: Without empathy, conflicts are more likely to escalate, as individuals are less inclined to seek understanding or compromise. This can create a tense and divisive workplace atmosphere. 4. *Lower team cohesion*: Teams lacking in empathy may struggle with collaboration and cohesion, as team members may feel undervalued or misunderstood. This can limit teamwork and the achievement of collective goals. 5. *Decreased morale and engagement*: A workplace characterised by low empathy can lead to decreased morale and employee engagement. Employees may feel disconnected, undervalued, and less motivated to contribute to their fullest potential.

5. *Positive work environment*: An empathetic workplace fosters a culture of mutual respect, understanding, and collaboration. This leads to higher job satisfaction, employee retention, and a supportive atmosphere.

Low Empathy in the Workplace

Conversely, when empathy is lacking in the workplace, negative behaviours and consequences can emerge:

1. *Miscommunication*: A lack of empathy often leads to misunderstandings and misinterpretations, as individuals may not fully consider the perspectives or emotional states of their colleagues or patients.

2. *Reduced patient satisfaction*: In healthcare settings, low empathy can result in patient care that feels impersonal, rushed, or uncaring. This can lead to decreased patient satisfaction and trust in healthcare providers.

3. *Increased conflict*: Without empathy, conflicts are more likely to escalate, as individuals are less inclined to seek understanding or compromise. This can create a tense and divisive workplace atmosphere.

4. *Lower team cohesion*: Teams lacking in empathy may struggle with collaboration and cohesion, as team members may feel undervalued or misunderstood. This can limit teamwork and the achievement of collective goals.

5. *Decreased morale and engagement*: A workplace characterised by low empathy can lead to decreased morale and employee engagement. Employees may feel disconnected, undervalued, and less motivated to contribute to their fullest potential.

Importance of Empathy in Dentistry

Empathy, a cornerstone of emotional intelligence, is profoundly important in dentistry, influencing the trajectory of dental professionals from their initial years as dental students through to the later stages of their careers. Empathy involves the ability to understand and share the feelings of another, an attribute that enhances personal well-being, patient care, and team dynamics. Its importance cannot be overstated, given the unique challenges and opportunities within dental practice. Below, we explore why empathy is vital at every stage of a dentist's career, examining its impact from personal, patient, and staff perspectives.

Dental Students

For dental students, developing empathy is crucial for personal growth. Empathy towards oneself and peers creates a supportive learning environment and aids in navigating the stress and pressure of dental education.

Early patient interactions provide a foundational understanding of the diverse needs and concerns that patients bring to the dental chair. Empathy allows students to build rapport with patients, enhancing communication and trust. These early experiences lay the groundwork for patient-centred care, highlighting the importance of understanding patients' fears, expectations, and experiences.

Collaborating with faculty and dental staff, students learn the importance of empathy in teamwork and leadership. Empathetic communication and understanding within the team facilitate smoother clinical operations and improve learning outcomes, setting the stage for effective team dynamics in future practice.

Early Career Dentists

As dentists transition into professional practice, empathy towards oneself remains critical, especially when facing the challenges of establishing a career, building a patient base, and navigating clinical responsibilities. Self-empathy fosters self-compassion, reducing the risk of burnout and promoting a healthy work-life balance.

For early career dentists, empathy deepens patient relationships, enhancing patient satisfaction and loyalty. By understanding and addressing patient anxieties and pain, dentists can alleviate fear, encouraging regular dental visits and adherence to treatment plans. This empathetic approach directly impacts growth reputation of the practice.

Developing empathetic relationships with staff and colleagues is essential for creating a positive workplace culture. Empathy facilitates effective communication, conflict resolution, and teamwork, contributing to a collaborative and supportive practice environment.

Mid-Career Dentists

Mid-career dentists, often juggling numerous professional and personal responsibilities, benefit immensely from self-empathy. Recognising one's own needs and limitations can help in setting realistic goals, prioritising self-care, and seeking support when needed.

At this stage, empathy enriches the dentist–patient relationship further, enabling dentists to provide highly personalised care. An empathetic understanding of the evolving needs of ageing patients, for instance, allows for adjustments in care plans and communication styles, enhancing patient engagement and treatment outcomes.

From the staff perspective, mid-career dentists who aspire to higher leadership positions within their practices or the wider dental community must recognise the critical importance of empathy when it comes to mentoring and guiding others. It promotes a culture of learning, shared objectives, and mutual respect, which in turn facilitates effective leadership.

Late Career Dentists

As dentists approach the later stages of their careers, empathy towards oneself can facilitate a smooth transition into retirement, acknowledging the emotional complexities of this life change. It allows for reflective practice, appreciating the successes and learning from the challenges of a long career. It also creates space to acknowledge the need for support at this stage from peers and colleagues who can guide and support.

Late career dentists, with years of experience, can leverage their deep empathetic insights to provide compassionate dental care in complex cases, navigate sensitive conversations about treatment options, and mentor younger dentists in the art of empathetic patient care.

From a leadership and legacy-building perspective, late career dentists play a pivotal role in imparting the values of empathy to the next generation of dental professionals. They have a lasting impact on practice culture and patient care standards by modelling empathetic conduct well beyond their retirement years.

Empathy and Litigation

Empathy in dentistry is not just a cornerstone of patient-centred care; it is also a strategic element in mitigating legal risks and avoiding litigation. This is one of the most significant stressors for dental professionals. The growing body of literature on medical malpractice shows a clear correlation between healthcare providers' empathetic engagement and a decrease in the incidence of legal actions by patients.

Empathy and Patient Satisfaction

The relationship between a dentist and their patient is central to successful outcomes. When dentists exhibit empathy, they create a more trusting and comfortable environment. Research has demonstrated that patients who perceive their healthcare providers as empathetic are more satisfied with their care, more likely to adhere to treatment plans, and less inclined to file complaints or pursue legal action (Beckman et al., 1994). Empathetic communication, characterised by active listening, acknowledgement of patients' concerns, and genuine expressions of care, can significantly alleviate patient anxiety, especially in a high-stress setting like dentistry, where fear and anxiety are prevalent (Hojat et al., 2011).

Empathy and Communication: A Legal Safety Net

Effective communication underpinned by empathy not only improves patient care but also serves as a preventive measure against misunderstandings that could lead to dissatisfaction and, ultimately, litigation. A landmark study by Levinson et al. (1997) revealed that surgeons who had never been sued spent more time in appointments and engaged more effectively with their patients compared to those who had experienced litigation. This underscores the importance of communication skills, including the ability to convey information clearly, listen actively, and respond to patients' emotional needs as critical components of empathetic care and legal risk management.

Understanding and Reducing Fear

Dental fear is a significant barrier to seeking and receiving dental care. An empathetic approach can help in understanding the root causes of a patient's fear, whether it's anxiety about pain, loss of control, or embarrassment about dental conditions. Dentists who are trained to recognise and address these fears can not only improve the patient experience but also mitigate the risk of complaints arising from misunderstandings or perceived neglect (Armfield et al., 2007).

Empathy Training Programmes

Given the clear benefits of empathy in reducing legal risks, incorporating empathy training into dental education and continuing professional development is crucial. Programmes that focus on developing communication skills, recognising non-verbal cues, and managing challenging conversations can equip dentists with the tools needed to build stronger, more empathetic relationships with their patients. Such training in medical research has been shown to enhance patient satisfaction, reduce the likelihood of litigation, and increase the overall quality of care (Riess et al., 2012).

The Role of Team Empathy

The empathetic quality of patient care is not solely the responsibility of the dentist; it extends to the entire dental team. Staff members who interact with patients, from receptionists to dental hygienists, play a crucial role in shaping the patient's overall experience. Training programmes that include the entire dental team can foster an empathetic practice culture, further reducing the likelihood of patient dissatisfaction and potential legal issues.

For dental practitioners, the threat of litigation is a significant source of stress, which can impact their well-being and the quality of care they provide. Cultivating an empathetic practice not only reduces this legal risk but also contributes to professional satisfaction. When dentists and their teams engage empathetically with patients, they not only create a positive environment for their patients but also for themselves, leading to reduced stress, higher job satisfaction, and a lower risk of burnout.

How to Develop Empathy?

Empathy in dentistry is not just a soft skill; it is a foundational aspect of providing compassionate, patient-centred care. Developing empathy can significantly enhance the patient experience, improve communication, and foster a positive workplace culture. Self-empathy, the ability to recognise and understand one's own emotions, is the first step toward cultivating empathy for others.

Below are suggestions to develop self-empathy as well as empathy with patients and staff.

Developing Self-Empathy in Dentistry

The journey of a dental professional is often marked by a unique set of challenges and stressors, ranging from patient anxiety management to the complex nature of dental procedures, not to mention the challenges of running a practice. Amid these demands, developing self-empathy becomes key for dentists to maintain their own well-being and enhance their ability to deliver compassionate care.

Self-empathy is the practice of treating oneself with the same kindness, concern, and support one would show to others, involving understanding one's own feelings and needs without judgement or criticism. It emphasises a compassionate and accepting approach to personal mistakes, shortcomings, and challenges. According to Neff (2003), self-empathy or self-compassion, comprises three main components: self-kindness, common humanity, and mindfulness. It enables individuals to maintain emotional equilibrium and fosters resilience in the face of adversity.

Self-empathy involves acknowledging one's feelings and needs without judgement. It is about allowing oneself to experience emotions fully, understand them, and respond with kindness and patience, similar to how one would treat a good friend. This practice is essential in dentistry, where perfectionism and high expectations can often lead to self-criticism and burnout.

Practical Ways to Develop Self-Empathy

- **Reflection and Mindfulness**
  Regular self-reflection is a powerful tool for developing self-empathy. Dentists can set aside time each day to reflect on their experiences, emotions, and reactions. This practice can help identify stressors and triggers, providing insights into how to cope with them more effectively. Getting into the habit of daily journalling for a few moments to "check in" with the emotional landscape can have a profound impact on well-being. Mindfulness meditation, a practice that encourages present-moment awareness without judgement, can complement self-reflection by helping dentists stay grounded and centred, even in stressful situations. According to a study by Shapiro et al. (2005), mindfulness-based stress reduction programmes significantly improve mental well-being in healthcare providers.

- **Peer Support Groups**
  Participating in peer support groups can also facilitate the development of self-empathy. These groups provide a safe space for sharing experiences, challenges, and successes, allowing dentists to realise they are not alone in their struggles. Peer support can foster a sense of community and belonging, which is vital for emotional resilience. A review by West et al. (2018) underscores the effectiveness of social support networks in reducing burnout and promoting well-being among medical professionals.

- **Developing a Growth Mindset**
  Embracing a growth mindset, where challenges are viewed as opportunities for learning and growth, can enhance self-empathy. Dentists should celebrate their achievements, however small, and view mistakes as learning opportunities rather than failures. Continuing education and professional development can reinforce this mindset by providing dentists with new skills and knowledge, thereby boosting their confidence and reducing feelings of inadequacy. Dweck (2006) highlights the benefits of a growth mindset in fostering resilience and self-compassion.

- **Setting Realistic Expectations**
  Dentists often set high standards for themselves, which can lead to disappointment and self-criticism when these are not met. By setting realistic expectations and recognising the limits of what can be achieved, dentists can reduce unnecessary pressure. This practice involves acknowledging that perfection is

unattainable and that making mistakes is a natural part of the learning process. A balanced, realistic approach to goal-setting can promote a healthier work-life balance and prevent burnout.

- **Professional Counselling/Therapy**
  Seeking professional counselling or therapy can be an effective way for dentists to develop self-empathy if they require deeper work to deal with ingrained behaviours from the past. Mental health professionals can provide strategies and tools at an individual level for managing stress, dealing with negative self-talk, and building emotional resilience. Counselling can offer a confidential and supportive environment to explore personal challenges and develop coping mechanisms.

Developing self-empathy is a continuous and evolving process that plays a critical role in the well-being and professional growth of dentists. By practising mindfulness, engaging in peer support, embracing a growth mindset, setting realistic expectations, and seeking professional help when needed, dentists can cultivate a compassionate and understanding relationship with themselves. This not only enhances their personal health but also empowers them to provide the highest level of care to their patients. As the dental profession continues to evolve, fostering self-empathy will remain a key factor in navigating the challenges and rewards of this demanding yet fulfilling career.

Enhancing Empathy with Patients

Empathy in dentistry is a critical component of effective patient care, enhancing patient satisfaction, compliance, and overall treatment outcomes. As dental professionals navigate the complexities of their careers, developing and nurturing empathy towards patients can profoundly impact their practice.

Empathy with patients involves understanding their fears, anxieties, and needs from their perspective, which can reduce patient stress and increase satisfaction with dental care (Levinson et al., 2010).

Much research demonstrates the importance of empathy in healthcare generally, with studies showing that empathetic practitioners can significantly improve patient satisfaction and treatment adherence (Hojat et al., 2011).

Practical Ways to Develop Empathy with Patients

1. **Active Listening**
   The foundation of empathy is active listening, which involves fully focusing on what the patient is saying, understanding their message, responding appropriately, and remembering the information. Active listening also means noticing non-verbal cues, such as body language and facial expressions. It requires being fully present and avoiding distractions to communication, increasingly difficult

as we live in an age of shrinking attention spans! Dentists can practice active listening by summarising what the patient has said and asking follow-up questions, thereby ensuring understanding and making the patient feel heard and valued.

2. **Empathy Training**
   Empathy is a muscle that can be developed! Participating in empathy training programmes can significantly enhance a dentist's ability to connect with patients. These programmes often include role-playing, reflective practice, and communication skills workshops. Such training helps dentists recognise and respond to patients' emotional states effectively. A systematic review by Kelm et al. (2014) found that empathy training could improve healthcare outcomes by enhancing provider–patient communication.

3. **Building Cultural Competence**
   Understanding and respecting cultural differences is crucial for developing empathy. Dentists should strive to build cultural competence by learning about the diverse backgrounds of their patients and understanding how cultural factors may influence patients' health beliefs and behaviours. This knowledge can foster a more inclusive environment, making patients from various cultural backgrounds feel understood and respected.

   Cultural competency equips dentists with the skills to navigate the linguistic and cultural barriers that might otherwise impede communication. For instance, certain cultures may view oral health differently or may have specific beliefs about health interventions. By understanding these perspectives, dentists can tailor their communication to ensure clarity and comprehension, thereby enhancing patient understanding and cooperation.

   Developing cultural competence is a dynamic and continuous process that enables dentists to provide effective care across diverse patient populations. Here are some practical ways for dentists to enhance their cultural competence:

   1. *Engage in Cultural Competency Training*
      - Participate in workshops and seminars focused on cultural sensitivity and competence.
      - Include staff in training sessions to ensure the whole team is culturally aware.

   2. *Learn about the Cultures of Your Patient Base*
      - Research and understand the cultural backgrounds, health beliefs, and practices of the communities you serve.
      - Use reliable sources and community resources for accurate and respectful understanding.

   3. *Improve Communication Skills*
      - Employ language interpretation services when necessary to overcome language barriers.
      - Learn basic greetings and phrases in the languages most commonly spoken by your patients.

4. *Foster an Inclusive Environment*
   - Display culturally diverse materials and signage in your office.
   - Ensure office policies are sensitive to cultural and religious needs, such as dietary restrictions or prayer times.

5. *Seek Feedback from Patients*
   - Use patient feedback to understand how well your practice meets the needs of diverse populations.
   - Implement changes based on feedback to improve cultural competence continually.

6. *Build Community Connections*
   - Collaborate with community leaders and organisations to gain insights into the cultural needs of the community.
   - Participate in community health events to engage with different cultural groups.

7. *Reflect on Personal Biases and Attitudes*
   - Regularly reflect on your own cultural biases and how they might affect patient care.
   - Commit to ongoing personal growth and understanding in cultural competence.

By integrating these practical steps into their practice, dentists can significantly enhance their cultural competence, leading to improved patient satisfaction, better healthcare outcomes, and a more inclusive dental care environment.

Trust is an essential element of the dentist–patient relationship. Patients are more likely to follow through with treatment recommendations and engage in preventive oral health behaviours when they trust their dentist. Cultural competency helps in building this trust by demonstrating respect for the patient's background, beliefs, and preferences. When patients feel understood and respected, they are more likely to disclose relevant health information, express concerns, and ask questions, all of which are critical for effective dental care and patient safety.

The importance of understanding diversity and cultural competency in dental practice cannot be overstated, as it significantly influences patient rapport, treatment compliance, and overall oral health outcomes.

1. **Patient-Centred Communication**

   Adopting a patient-centred approach to communication involves focusing on the patient's individual needs, preferences, and values. This method encourages dentists to explore the patient's perspective, involve them in decision-making, and provide personalised care. Strategies include using layman's terms instead of medical jargon, ensuring the patient understands their treatment options, and showing genuine interest in their concerns and questions.

2. Reflective Practice

Reflective practice involves regularly reflecting on one's interactions with patients and the emotional aspects of care. By taking time to reflect on their experiences, dentists can gain insights into their strengths and areas for improvement when it comes to their levels of empathy with patients. Reflective practice can be facilitated through journalling, peer discussions, or mentorship programmes, allowing dentists to develop a deeper understanding of their patients' experiences and how to enhance the empathetic quality of care.

Developing empathy with patients is a dynamic and ongoing process that requires conscious effort, reflection, and adaptation. By actively listening, engaging in empathy training, building cultural competence, practising patient-centred communication, reflecting on personal experiences, maintaining emotional well-being, and fostering a supportive team environment, dentists can enhance their ability to connect with patients on a deeper level. This empathetic approach not only improves patient satisfaction and outcomes but also enriches the professional and personal fulfilment of dental practitioners. As the field of dentistry continues to evolve, the emphasis on empathy will remain a cornerstone of patient-centred care, underlining the profound impact of understanding, compassion, and connection in the healing process.

Developing Empathy with Staff

Creating a culture of empathy within the dental team not only improves staff satisfaction and retention but also enhances the overall patient experience. Developing empathy within the dental practice, particularly towards staff, is a critical component of creating a positive high performing, and harmonious work environment. Empathy, the ability to understand and share the feelings of another, is not just a foundational element of patient care but is equally important in interpersonal relationships among dental practice staff. When dentists actively cultivate empathy towards their team, they set a tone of respect, support, and collaboration that can significantly enhance team cohesion, job satisfaction, and ultimately, the quality of patient care. Below are some key ways to develop empathy with colleagues:

- **Build a Culture of Open Communication**
  - *Encourage regular feedback*: Create an environment where staff feel comfortable providing feedback without fear of reprisal. Regular team meetings and one-on-one sessions can provide platforms for open dialogue, allowing team members to express concerns, share ideas, and offer suggestions for improvement. This practice not only helps in addressing issues but also in understanding the perspectives and emotional states of team members (Edmondson, 1999).
  - *Active listening*: Practice active listening to each team member by giving full attention to the speaker, acknowledging their thoughts and feelings,

and responding thoughtfully. This approach not only fosters open communication but also helps in understanding the underlying issues or concerns staff may have.

- **Recognising and Addressing Burnout**
  - *Monitor workloads*: Keep an eye on the workloads of staff to prevent burnout. Overworked employees can experience decreased job satisfaction and productivity, leading to a negative work environment.
  - *Promote work-life balance*: Encourage staff to maintain a healthy work-life balance by offering flexible working hours where possible and respecting their time off. Recognising the importance of personal time can significantly improve morale and job satisfaction.

- **Fostering Team Collaboration**
  - *Team-building/Social activities*: Engage in team-building and social activities that are not only fun but also help in breaking down barriers between staff members and between staff and dentists. These activities can improve understanding and empathy by allowing everyone to see each other in a different light, outside of the professional setting.

- **Practising Empathy in Leadership**
  - *Lead by example*: Demonstrate empathy in your actions and interactions. Being approachable, showing genuine concern for staff well-being, and actively supporting their professional development can inspire similar behaviour among team members. Consider the impacts of decisions on staff and involve them in the decision-making process when appropriate. This approach not only demonstrates empathy but also empowers staff and can lead to more effective and inclusive solutions.

- **Supporting Professional Development**
  - *Individual development plans*: Work with staff to create individual professional development plans. Recognising and supporting their career aspirations can lead to higher levels of job satisfaction and loyalty, particularly among the younger generations. Showing an interest in individual professional development shows empathy and understanding of the individual's ambitions.

By integrating these practical approaches, dentists can foster an environment of empathy and understanding within their practices, leading to a more cohesive and supportive team. Empathy towards staff not only enhances the work environment but also indirectly benefits patient care, making it an essential skill for dentists to develop and nurture throughout their careers.

Conclusion

Throughout the stages of a dental career, empathy serves as a guiding principle for personal growth, patient treatment, and professional connections.

From the formative years of dental education to the reflective moments of a late career, empathy enriches the dental profession by fostering meaningful connections, enhancing patient trust and satisfaction, and building collaborative, supportive teams. Its significance extends beyond clinical abilities, representing the essence of dental practice.

As the dental profession continues to evolve, the timeless value of empathy remains constant, underscoring its critical role in shaping compassionate, patient-centred care, and nurturing supportive workplace environments.

EMPATHY: DENTAL PRACTITIONER PERSPECTIVE

CIARA SCOTT

Introduction

Empathy has been described as the ability to understand another person's thoughts, feelings and point of view. Empathy allows us to step away from our own perspective and "walk in another person's shoes."

Many people who choose professions like dentistry do so because we want to build caring relationships in our professional practice. As inexperienced practitioners, we are naturally focused on what we need to do in patient interactions. It would seem to follow that as we gain skills, experience and confidence, we would also build the capacity for empathy. However, research suggests that empathy scores can decline during clinical training, a trend also seen in medical practitioners (Yarascavitch et al., 2009). Additionally, a recent study reported that patients considered chatbot responses to an online medical forum up to 10 times more empathetic and informative that those written by medical practitioners (Ayers et al., 2023). It follows that like the other skills and techniques we use in our practice, empathy is something we can continue to build awareness of and experience of how we use it in our personal and professional relationships and also of when we can overuse empathy.

Like other healthcare professions, much of the focus on training in dental schools traditionally promoted the acquisition of knowledge and technical skills. A shift towards models of patient-centred care places greater emphasis on communication skills, recognising that technical skills contribute to only a percentage of success at work. Emerging science in this field supports us to understand why and how to apply this. While we may all have different definitions of professional success, be it engagement, enjoyment, patient outcomes, profitability, reputation or a combination of these, our emotional capital and our ability to use empathy appropriately and effectively contributes significantly to how we manage our relationships at work and our stress, both through success and during setbacks.

It's valuable to recognise that while professional training primarily focuses on individual competence, it cannot be assumed that groups of individually competent professionals who work together will become competent teams (Lingard, 2009). There is a complex interplay of how individuals bring their skills, knowledge, and experience to work and share responsibility for success and setbacks to create a culture of collective competence. Building emotional capital at work supports patients, professionals and ultimately population health. When we bring awareness to challenging situations and reflect on difficult interactions, we can improve our relationships at work with ourselves, our patients and our colleagues, positively impacting on our engagement, fulfilment, risk of burnout and not least importantly, the bottom line. There is a common

DOI: 10.1201/9781003379829-9

business analogy that 10% of your clients cause 90% of your problems. Empathy is at the core of how we understand and appreciate others to build positive relationships in our practices with our patients, our staff or our colleagues. The 10% of our practice that's a thorn in our side can become less of a burden. Empathy is inextricably linked with trust, respect and psychological safety at work.

What Is Empathy?

The Oxford English Dictionary defines empathy as "the ability to understand and appreciate another person's feelings, experience, etc." Its earliest use in the English language was in psychological theory and there have been subtle shifts in meaning through the decades. Empathy can be described as cognitive (something we know), affective or emotional (something we feel) and behavioural (something we do). While some practitioners may have natural empathy in how they interact with patients and colleagues, empathy can also be learnt and practised. We can also overuse or misuse empathy. While there are similarities, empathy can sometimes be confused with the concepts of sympathy, compassion, and caring.

Simply, sympathy is something that we express – our own thoughts and feelings about another person's feelings or situation. However, empathy is not about ourselves but is the ability to recognise, acknowledge, and respond to another person's perspective. While empathy is often cited as a valued trait in practitioners that is positively correlated with improved patient satisfaction and improved outcomes, the real measure of empathy is how it is perceived and felt by the other person.

Caring has been described as "a simple process, cherished by professionals, but as a lived experience it can be more complex" (Shanahan, 2020). Shein (2009) also provides rich insights into the complexity of "helping relationships" and why helping is not always "helpful." While there can be a hierarchy in a sympathetic relationships and caring relationships, there is equality in an empathetic relationship, building rapport, trust and recognition of other perspectives. If sympathy is giving, then empathic relationships create the space to listen to others. Importantly, being empathic is not the same as being agreeable. Practising empathy allows us to listen respectfully and acknowledge different perspectives. We can be empathetic while also maintaining our own professional judgement and perspectives.

The shift towards patient-centred approaches to care has led to a plethora of courses and books promoting communication skills. Many of these have a deficit approach, focusing on managing risk and complaints, while others emphasise positive incentives, such as ethical sales.

This chapter focuses on why learning and practising empathy will support happier professional lives and more successful professional relationships. The field of positive organisational scholarship focuses on the behaviours, dynamics, and cultures that lead to optimal functioning at work. Empathy is at the centre of social connectedness and affects our relationships with staff, patients, and colleagues, whether you're leading a team or working within one. There is a correlation between self-evaluated empathy and leadership behaviour. More importantly, leadership effectiveness is associated more strongly with leadership behaviours rather than individual traits such as empathy (Skinner and Spurgeon, 2005). Thus, learning how to use empathy appropriately is more important than believing we are empathetic.

We have already explained the power differential that can exist in sympathetic and caring relationships. This power imbalance can also exist in our professional relationships; between dentist and patient, between dentist and nurse, between practice manager and patient. Clinical training often involves instruction, direction, supervision, judgement, feedback and assessment. As we normalise this workplace culture and style of learning and communicating, we can often consciously and unconsciously bring this to other professional relationships. Even in the context of patient-centred care, our professional training has set us up to be experts in our field and the professional dynamic exists where patients will seek help and advice and we will share our expertise. This dynamic of help seeking and telling can be at dissonance with true empathy.

In one study of primary care medical consultations, in an average 15-minute consultation, the doctor did 80% of the speaking and, during this time, asked closed questions and offered advice and instructions. Active patient participation in consultations depends on a complex interplay of patient, practitioner and contextual factors, but supportive conversation styles that include praise, reassurance, and empathy encourage active patient participation (Street et al., 2005). Empathy enables us to flatten traditional hierarchies in healthcare relationships and acknowledge that while the dentist is an expert in their field, the patient is also an expert in their own health, the dental nurse is an expert in their own field, and so on. Thus, through building empathy, trust, and respect in positive professional relationships, all team members flourish and contribute to patient-centred practice. There is evidence that using language that builds respect and supports autonomy can be effective in reducing hierarchies in clinical settings and improving outcomes (Burke et al., 2022). We can also be aware that anxiety can heighten the perception of control rather than support; this means that some patients may not perceive empathy or support even when we offer it or intend it and an awareness of this can support patients who find dental settings difficult.

Conversely, a lack of empathy and depersonalisation have been identified as causes of burnout.

When we do not feel trusted or valued in our professional relationships, this can play a significant role in our engagement, job satisfaction, and retention and also impact on how we manage communicate, manage conflict, quality, and patient safety and patient outcomes and risk. Research suggests that dentists can lose empathy as their career progresses and become more cynical, so building awareness of when we are at risk of this and may benefit from a break or more support is valuable.

Equally, it is possible to overuse empathy. Emotional empathy impacts on our own feelings and affective empathy is a term used to describe when we absorb other people's emotions. It is important that as we practice empathy, that we manage our own boundaries so that in practising empathy in caring relationship we are not absorbing negative emotions and stress that others may share with us.

Empathy is at the core of building positive relationships and positive connections. With empathy, we can listen and be curious, others feel genuinely valued, building capacity for collaboration. This is the essence of patient-centred care and shared decision-making. Without this positive connection from empathy, our working relationships be transactional and questions can feel more like interrogation rather than curiosity.

Even within the sphere of evidence-based practice, we can have different perspectives and preferences for techniques and treatments. The evidence base does not provide one-size-fits-all solutions. Empathy supports us to respect and value difference and build curiosity about difference. Rather than judging, empathy enables us to be open to and curious about other's perspectives, enabling decision-making, empowering professional relationships and creating opportunities for learning.

Case Study

Jo was top in her graduating class and was delighted to accept a role working in a large specialist orthodontic practice. She had two periods of maternity leave very soon after she qualified and has recently returned to work to a full book of transfer cases. She's still getting used to the practice, the team, and the patients, as well as getting used to new childcare arrangements at home.

She entered the principal's office one lunchtime, visibly distressed:

> Can I ask your advice about child A's case? You planned her treatment last year, but it's a really difficult case and I'm not sure it's going well. The child became really upset during the last two visits. Her mum just called the practice to tell me that she has no confidence in me and doesn't want me to look after her daughter anymore. They have an appointment with me this afternoon, but she's demanded to be transferred back to you.

The Principal, Marion, reassured her: "You're a great orthodontist, don't let her upset you. This will be a great opportunity for you to learn."

"But she doesn't want me to see her child!"

"It wouldn't be appropriate for me to step in; you've got this. I trust that you can handle this."

Jo left the office. Another orthodontist, Caroline, who had overheard some of the interaction met Jo later in the restroom. Jo was in tears. Caroline was 10 years older than Jo and still remembered the stress of sleepless nights and full diaries of patients: "Can I help?"

Jo and Caroline spent the rest of their lunch break going through the case records, the treatment progress, the parent's concerns, and the potential options. Caroline was not Jo's line manager, so she didn't want to overstep or undermine Jo's confidence. She listened with empathy and tried to support Jo's decision. She agreed to see the child A and her mum on top of her scheduled patients to support a resolution. The child managed the appointment well and the mum was happy. Caroline reassured child A and her mum that the treatment was progressing well, but understood it was a very challenging case. Jo told Caroline she was a lifesaver. Caroline was happy that she had been able to help Jo, the child, and her mum; it was a good day.

That evening, Caroline shared some of her day with her husband over dinner. She told him how she had been happy to help Jo and resolve of the issue, and also that she was annoyed with Marion.

"You seem overwhelmed; I can feel the stress just listening to you," he said.

Summary

While Karen wanted to support Jo's autonomy and encourage her to learn through experience, her response lacked empathy. If she had created the space to become aware of Jo's distress, she would have recognised that positive soundbites were not the solution and Jo really needed to feel listened to without judgement and supported to regain professional confidence. When we lack professional confidence or competence, purely facilitative approaches are less useful.

However, Caroline's awareness of Jo's distress affected her. Rather than dissipating the stress, Caroline absorbed it and brought it home with her. This is affective empathy. When we practice empathy, it is useful to bring awareness of our role in another person's story and how we manage our own boundaries.

References

Armfield JM, Stewart JF, Spencer AJ. (2007). The vicious cycle of dental fear: exploring the interplay between oral health, service utilization and dental fear. *BMC Oral Health*, 7, 1.

Ayers JW, Poliak A, Dredze M, Leas EC, Zhu Z, Kelley JB, et al. (2023). Comparing physician and artificial intelligence chatbot responses to patient questions posted to a public social media forum. *JAMA Intern Med*, 183(6), 589–596.

Beckman HB, Markakis KM, Suchman AL, Frankel RM. (1994). The doctor-patient relationship and malpractice: Lessons from plaintiff depositions. *Arch Intern Med*, 154(12), 1365–1370.

Burke TJ, Young VJ, Duggan A. (2022). Recognizing the blurred boundary between health-related support and control in close relationships. *Pers Relat*, 29(4), 644–673.

Dweck CS. (2006). *Mindset: The New Psychology of Success*. Random House.

Edmondson A. (1999). Psychological safety and learning behavior in work teams. *Administrative Sci Q*, 44(2), 350–383.

Hojat M, Louis DZ, Markham FW, Wender R, Rabinowitz C, Gonnella JS. (2011). Physicians' empathy and clinical outcomes for diabetic patients. *Acad Med*, 86(3), 359–364.

Kadanakuppe S. (2015). Effective communication and empathy skills in dentistry for better dentist-patient relationships. *J Dent Probl Solut*, 2(3), 058–059.

Kelm Z, Womer J, Walter JK, Feudtner C. (2014). Interventions to cultivate physician empathy: A systematic review. *BMC Med Educ*, 14, 219.

Levinson W, Roter DL, Mullooly JP, Dull VT, Frankel RM. (1997). Physician-patient communication. The relationship with malpractice claims among primary care physicians and surgeons. *JAMA*, *277*(7), 553–559.

Lingard L. (2009). What we see and don't see when we look at "competence": Notes on a God term. *Adv Health Sci Educ*, *14*(5), 625–628.

Levinson W, Lesser CS, Epstein RM. (2010). Developing physician communication skills for patient-centered care. *Health Aff*, *29*(7), 1310–1318.

Narang R, Mittal L, Saha S, Aggarwal VP, Sood P, Mehra S. (2019). Empathy among dental students: A systematic review of literature. *J Indian Soc Pedod Prev Dent*, *37*(4), 316–326.

Nash DA. (2010). Ethics, empathy, and the education of dentists. *J Dent Educ*, *74*(6), 567–578.

Neff KD. (2003). Self-compassion: An alternative conceptualization of a healthy attitude toward oneself. *Self Identity*, *2*(2), 85–101.

Riess H, Kelley JM, Bailey RW, Dunn EJ, Phillips M. (2012). Empathy training for resident physicians: A randomized controlled trial of A neuroscience-informed curriculum. *J Gen Intern Med*, *27*(10), 1280–1286.

Shanahan F. (2020). *The language of illness*. Liberties Press.

Shapiro SL, Astin JA, Bishop SR, Cordova M. (2005). Mindfulness-based stress reduction for health care professionals: Results from a randomized trial. *Int J Stress Manage*, *12*(2), 164–176.

Shein EH. (2009). *Helping*. Berrett Koehler Publishers.

Skinner C, Spurgeon P. (2005). Valuing empathy and emotional intelligence in health leadership: A study of empathy, leadership behaviours and outcome effectiveness. *Health Serv Manage Res*, *18*(1), 1–12.

Street RL, Gordon HS, Ward MM, Krupat E, Kravitz RL. (2005). Patient participation in medical consultations: Why some patients are more involved than others. *Med Care*, *43*(10), 960–969.

West CP, Dyrbye LN, Shanafelt TD. (2018). Physician burnout: Contributors, consequences and solutions. *J Intern Med*, *283*(6), 516–529.

Yarascavitch C, Regehr G, Hodges B, Haas DA. (2009). Changes in dental student empathy during training. *J Dent Educ*, *73*(4), 509–517.

6

EQ CRITICAL SKILL IV

Relationship Skills

MARY COLLINS

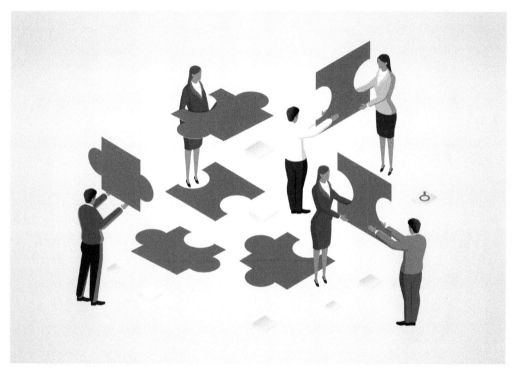

(*Source*: https://www.gettyimages.co.uk/detail/illustration/build-new-teams-to-develop-new-business-royalty-free-illustration/1456477620)

Introduction

Plato, the Greek philosopher and student of Socrates, offered profound insights into various aspects of life, including the importance of relationships. One quote that describes his view on the depth and significance of connections between individuals is: "Every heart sings a song, incomplete, until another heart whispers back. Those who wish to sing always find a song. At the touch of a lover, everyone becomes a poet."

This quote encapsulates the transformative power of relationships, suggesting that it is in connection with others that we find completion, expression, and the inspiration to create and live fully.

DOI: 10.1201/9781003379829-10

This chapter will focus on the following topics:

- Definition of relationship skills in emotional intelligence
- Importance of relationship skills in dentistry
- How to develop relationship skills
- Dental practitioner perspective

Definition of Relationship Skills in Emotional Intelligence

Relationship skills in the context of emotional intelligence (EI) refer to the capacity to manage, influence, and inspire interactions with others effectively. This competency is foundational for building positive, constructive relationships both in personal and professional settings. It encompasses a range of abilities such as clear communication, active listening, conflict resolution, empathy, and the ability to inspire and influence others positively. These skills are vital for anyone looking to lead, collaborate, or simply maintain healthy relationships with others.

The RocheMartin definition of relationship skills, as part of their Emotional Capital Report (ECR), emphasizes the strategic development of one's interpersonal skills to build and maintain strong, effective relationships. According to RocheMartin, relationship skills in EI involve the adeptness at inducing desirable responses in others. This means not only being able to communicate effectively but also being capable of inspiring and persuading others toward a common goal, demonstrating empathy and understanding, and managing conflicts or disagreements in a way that strengthens relationships rather than weakens them (**Table 6.1**).

Characteristics of High Levels of Relationship Skills

- *Effective communication*: Individuals with high relationship skills communicate clearly, ensuring that their message is understood as intended. They are also excellent listeners, showing genuine interest in others' opinions and feedback, which fosters an atmosphere of open dialogue and collaboration.
- *Empathy and understanding*: Empathy is the ability to understand and share the feelings of another. In the workplace, this translates to recognizing the emotions and perspectives of colleagues and responding appropriately. Such individuals can navigate sensitive situations with grace, providing support when needed and contributing to a positive work environment.
- *Conflict resolution*: Conflict is inevitable in any workplace, but those with high relationship skills can manage disagreements constructively. They approach conflicts with a problem-solving mindset, seeking solutions that acknowledge everyone's needs and preserve the integrity of professional relationships.
- *Building and maintaining relationships*: People with strong relationship skills are adept at building networks within the organization. They maintain these relationships through regular, meaningful interactions, helping to create a cohesive and supportive work environment.

Table 6.1   Relationship Skills: Behaviors of High and Low Levels in the Workplace

HIGH RELATIONSHIP SKILLS: BEHAVIORS AT WORK	LOW RELATIONSHIP SKILLS: BEHAVIORS AT WORK
When someone possesses high levels of relationship skills, we see the following characteristics in their behavior and interactions:	When someone possesses low levels of relationship skills, we see the following characteristics in their behavior and interactions:
1. *Effective communication*: Individuals with high relationship skills communicate clearly, ensuring that their message is understood as intended. They are also excellent listeners, showing genuine interest in others' opinions and feedback, which fosters an atmosphere of open dialogue and collaboration.	1. *Poor communication*: In contrast, low levels of relationship skills often manifest in poor communication, including unclear messaging, frequent misunderstandings, and a lack of effective listening. This can lead to confusion, errors, and inefficiencies within teams.
2. *Empathy and understanding*: Empathy is the ability to understand and share the feelings of another. In the workplace, this translates to recognizing the emotions and perspectives of colleagues and responding appropriately. Such individuals can navigate sensitive situations with grace, providing support when needed and contributing to a positive work environment.	2. *Lack of empathy*: A deficiency in empathy can result in an inability to connect with colleagues on a personal level, making it difficult to build trust and rapport. This can create a cold or impersonal work environment, where employees feel undervalued and disengaged.
3. *Conflict resolution*: Conflict is inevitable in any workplace, but those with high relationship skills can manage disagreements constructively. They approach conflicts with a problem-solving mindset, seeking solutions that acknowledge everyone's needs and preserve the integrity of professional relationships.	3. *Ineffective conflict management*: Without the ability to resolve conflicts constructively, minor disagreements can escalate, damaging relationships and team morale. Individuals with low relationship skills may avoid addressing conflicts directly or, conversely, handle them in a confrontational manner, both of which can be detrimental.
4. *Building and maintaining relationships*: People with strong relationship skills are adept at building networks within the organization. They maintain these relationships through regular, meaningful interactions, helping to create a cohesive and supportive work environment.	4. *Difficulty in building relationships*: People with low relationship skills often struggle to form or maintain professional relationships. This isolation can hinder collaboration and limit opportunities for personal and career development.
5. *Influencing and persuading*: Influencing others toward a common goal is a hallmark of high relationship skills. These individuals can rally a team, motivate colleagues, and drive projects forward with enthusiasm and conviction, ensuring team alignment and commitment.	5. *Poor influence*: A lack of persuasive ability means that these individuals may struggle to inspire or motivate teams, leading to a lack of direction, commitment, and enthusiasm for projects.

- *Influencing and persuading*: Influencing others toward a common goal is a hallmark of high relationship skills. These individuals can rally a team, motivate colleagues, and drive projects forward with enthusiasm and conviction, ensuring team alignment and commitment.

Characteristics of Low Levels of Relationship Skills

- *Poor communication*: In contrast, low levels of relationship skills often manifest in poor communication, including unclear messaging, frequent misunderstandings, and a lack of effective listening. This can lead to confusion, errors, and inefficiencies within teams.

- *Lack of empathy*: A deficiency in empathy can result in an inability to connect with colleagues on a personal level, making it difficult to build trust and rapport. This can create a cold or impersonal work environment, where employees feel undervalued and disengaged.

- *Ineffective conflict management*: Without the ability to resolve conflicts constructively, minor disagreements can escalate, damaging relationships and team morale. Individuals with low relationship skills may avoid addressing conflicts directly or, conversely, handle them in a confrontational manner, both of which can be detrimental.
- *Difficulty in building relationships*: People with low relationship skills often struggle to form or maintain professional relationships. This isolation can hinder collaboration and limit opportunities for personal and career development.
- *Poor influence*: A lack of persuasive ability means that these individuals may struggle to inspire or motivate teams, leading to a lack of direction, commitment, and enthusiasm for projects.

Importance of Relationship Skills in Dentistry

Developing relationship skills is crucial for dentists throughout their career trajectory, from dental school to retirement. These skills, which encompass effective communication, empathy, conflict resolution, and teamwork, are not static; they evolve and adapt to meet the changing demands of each career stage. The importance of honing these skills at every career juncture cannot be overstated, as they directly impact patient care, workplace dynamics, professional growth, and personal fulfilment.

Dental Student

For dental students, relationship skills are foundational to their education and early clinical experiences. Learning to communicate effectively with patients, peers, and instructors is crucial. Dental education not only involves acquiring technical skills but also understanding patients' needs and concerns. Effective communication and empathy can enhance patient comfort, leading to better clinical outcomes and more fulfilling educational experiences. Studies have shown that empathy in dental students is associated with better patient satisfaction and can be improved with targeted training (Sherman and Cramer, 2005).

Practical approach:

- Engage in role-playing exercises to simulate patient interactions.
- Seek feedback from peers and mentors on communication and interpersonal skills.
- Participate in interprofessional education programs to understand and collaborate with other healthcare professionals.

Early Career

As dentists transition into their early careers, relationship skills become even more critical. They must navigate the complexities of working within a dental practice, managing staff, and building a patient base. Effective communication and leadership skills are essential for establishing trust with patients and colleagues. Furthermore, early-career dentists often face challenges such as dealing with difficult patients or managing the expectations of more experienced staff. Developing strong conflict resolution skills can mitigate these challenges and foster a positive work environment.

Practical approach:

- Attend workshops or seminars focused on leadership and communication in healthcare.
- Seek mentorship from experienced dentists to navigate early career challenges.
- Invest time in team-building activities to enhance collaboration and morale within the practice.

Mid-Career

Mid-career dentists, often with established practices and significant professional responsibilities, must continue to refine their relationship skills to navigate the evolving healthcare landscape. At this stage, mentoring younger dentists and dental students becomes an important role, requiring advanced communication, empathy, and leadership skills. Furthermore, mid-career professionals might engage in more complex patient cases or navigate changes within their practice, requiring a sophisticated understanding of patient psychology and staff management.

Practical approach:

- Participate in continuing education courses that focus not only on clinical skills but also on practice management and interpersonal communication.
- Serve as a mentor or instructor, which can further develop empathy and leadership abilities.
- Lead by example, demonstrating effective relationship skills in every interaction, thereby setting a standard for the practice.

Late Career to Retirement

As dentists approach late career and consider retirement, relationship skills take on new dimensions. Transitioning patients to other dentists, advising dental practices, or engaging in community health initiatives can all benefit from honed relationship skills. Moreover, late-career dentists often hold positions of influence within professional associations or community groups, where they can advocate for the profession and mentor the next generation.

Practical approach:

- Engage in legacy-building activities, such as creating scholarships, participating in community health outreach, or writing about their experiences and insights.

- Actively participate in professional dental associations to influence policy and education, leveraging their relationship skills to foster change.
- Mentor young dentists not only in clinical skills but also in the art of building and maintaining professional relationships.

The development of relationship skills is a lifelong journey for dentists, crucial at every stage of their career. These skills are essential for providing excellent patient care, managing successful practices, navigating professional challenges, and achieving personal growth. Through intentional development and refinement of relationship skills, dentists can navigate the complexities of their profession at any stage, ultimately enriching their practice, their relationships, and their personal fulfilment.

How to Develop Relationship Skills

Developing relationship skills in dentistry is essential for success and fulfilment in the profession. These skills, vital at a personal level, patient level, and staff level encompass communication, empathy, leadership, and teamwork. Cultivating such skills can significantly enhance patient care, workplace dynamics, and personal well-being. This comprehensive approach involves practical strategies that can be implemented at each level.

Personal Level

- *Self-awareness and self-reflection*: The foundation of strong relationship skills begins with self-awareness. Dentists should engage in regular self-reflection to understand their communication style, emotional responses, and areas for growth. Tools like journaling or feedback from trusted colleagues can provide valuable insights into personal strengths and weaknesses.
- *Continuous learning*: Attending workshops, seminars, and courses focused on communication, leadership, and personal development can provide dentists with the tools and knowledge to improve their relationship skills. Psychometric profiles like the Emotional Capital Framework (ECR) can provide a measure of levels of relationship skills and suggestions to improve this important competence.
- *Work with a coach/mentor*: Having regular sessions with a coach or mentor on evaluating current levels of relationship skills and also identify how to enhance this area can be very impactful at a personal level.
- *Mentorship and peer support*: Engaging in mentorship, either as a mentor or mentee, and participating in peer support groups can provide valuable opportunities for learning and growth. These relationships offer a platform for sharing experiences, challenges, and strategies for developing relationship skills.
- *Networking and professional involvement*: Becoming involved in professional organizations, attending conferences, and networking with other dental professionals can expand one's perspective on relationship-building within the

profession. These interactions can introduce new ideas, strategies, and best practices for enhancing relationship skills.

Patient Level

- *Effective communication*: Clear and compassionate communication is essential for building positive relationships with patients. This involves not only explaining treatments and procedures clearly but also actively listening to patients' concerns and questions. Techniques such as "teach-back" method, where patients repeat back the information in their own words, can ensure understanding and foster a sense of involvement in their care (Ha and Longnecker, 2010).
- *Empathy*: Empathy and relationship skills go hand in hand. In many respects, empathy is "the root" of the relationship. Demonstrating empathy requires dentists to genuinely understand and share the feelings of their patients. This can be achieved by being present during interactions, acknowledging patients' anxieties or fears, and responding with kindness and reassurance. Training in empathic communication can improve patient satisfaction and compliance (Riess, 2017).
- *Patient-centred care*: Having an intentional patient-centred approach means considering patients' individual needs, preferences, and values in their care. Involving patients in decision-making, respecting their autonomy, and tailoring dental services to meet their specific needs can enhance the patient-dentist relationship.

Staff Level

- *Leadership and team-building*: Developing positive relationships at work requires effective leadership. This involves more than just managing a dental practice; it's about inspiring, motivating, and guiding staff toward shared goals. Regular team meetings, open communication channels, and collaborative decision-making processes can strengthen team cohesion and morale which leads to a better patient experience.
- *Conflict resolution*: Conflicts are inevitable in any workplace, in fact, healthy conflict is a factor in high-performance teams (Lencioni, 2002). How conflict is managed can significantly impact staff relationships. Adopting a proactive approach to conflict resolution, which involves listening to all parties, identifying underlying issues, and working collaboratively toward a solution, can prevent minor disagreements from escalating into major problems.
- *Recognition and development*: Acknowledging staff achievements, providing regular constructive feedback, and supporting their professional development are key aspects of building positive relationships. Encouraging staff to pursue further training and offering opportunities for career advancement can foster a supportive and motivated work environment.

Developing relationship skills in dentistry requires a multifaceted approach, addressing personal development, patient care, and staff management. By implementing practical strategies at each level, dentists can enhance their ability to build strong, positive relationships that contribute to professional success, patient satisfaction, and a harmonious work environment. Continuous learning, self-reflection, effective communication, and empathy are key components in this ongoing process.

Conclusion

The contrast between high and low levels of relationship skills in the workplace underscores the profound impact these competencies have on organizational culture and success. High levels of relationship skills contribute to a positive, productive work environment where individuals feel valued, understood, and motivated. On the other hand, low relationship skills can lead to a range of negative outcomes, including poor communication, unresolved conflicts, and a lack of team cohesion. As such, investing in the development of relationship skills across all levels of an organization is not just beneficial but essential for fostering a thriving, collaborative, and resilient workplace.

The RocheMartin model suggests that developing these relationship skills is not an innate talent but a set of competencies that can be learned and improved over time. By focusing on EI, individuals can enhance their ability to connect with others, navigate social complexities, and lead more effectively.

In the workplace, for instance, managers with high EI and strong relationship skills can foster a positive, productive environment, leading to improved team performance and job satisfaction. In personal contexts, these skills contribute to healthier, more fulfilling relationships, allowing individuals to communicate more effectively, resolve conflicts amicably, and deepen connections with those around them.

Relationship skills are a critical component of EI that enable individuals to build, maintain, and enhance relationships in both personal and professional spheres. According to RocheMartin, developing these skills involves a strategic approach to understanding and influencing the emotional dynamics of interactions, emphasizing the importance of empathy, communication, conflict resolution, and the ability to inspire and persuade others. By cultivating these skills, individuals can significantly improve their interactions and relationships, leading to greater personal and professional success.

RELATIONSHIP SKILLS: DENTAL PRACTITIONER PERSPECTIVE

PAUL O'DWYER

Why Are Relationships Important for a Successful Career in Dentistry?

From the outset, at the training stage, the colleagues and friends we meet at dental school are among the first important professional relationships we form. These are often lifelong and usually provide the foundation of our professional lives. By maintaining healthy respectful and nurturing professional relationships, they represent both a sounding board and a key support in the clinical practice of dentistry. Many dental schools train dentists in conjunction with other allied oral healthcare professionals including dental nurses, hygienists, therapists, and others. This not only exposes each trainee to the other elements/actors of the profession but plants the seeds for fruitful professional relationships into the future.

In thinking about the importance of relationships in a dental career, the key cornerstone of each practice is the relationship among the clinical team. Dentistry is ultimately patient-driven but team-delivered.

It is therefore self-evident that the trust factor among the treating clinical staff is both paramount and sacrosanct – built from strong high-quality relationships. These critical relationships are of over-arching value to the team and to clinical service delivery.

Building this good team **around** the clinician is often cited as advantageous. However, I would suggest that building a good team **with** the clinician is a more useful viewpoint. We know from the literature that high-quality relationships provide many benefits including the ability to "bounce back" better, achieve more, and strengthen a sense of purpose.

Engaged, motivated, and empathic team members raise quality of care, promote staff well-being, and are often vital factors to longer-term staff retention.

What Are the Key Relationships from Your Experience?

During undergraduate training, we are rightly instructed that the needs of the patient are placed at the centre of treatment planning and delivery. The treatment plan is primarily formed from an accurate, comprehensive, and definitive history. All clinicians will agree that this initial history usually represents both a clinical opportunity and usually represents the initial meeting of the dentist and patient. The importance of the history is not just from this clinical provision viewpoint but also as a starting point in the dentist–patient relationship.

The old adage of "You never get a second chance to make a good first impression" rings true. Trust between dentist and patient is often quickly formed from a warm, welcoming, and engaged clinician who attentively listens to the presenting complaint.

DOI: 10.1201/9781003379829-11

And while, we, as clinicians, are often primarily concerned with both the cause of the presenting issue and its potential treatment, we are also guided by the knowledge, that a trusting and engaged relationship, once formed, enhances patient outcomes, builds confidence, and maximizes compliance in our clinical instructions and directions.

General dentistry often sees patients attend infrequently. Typically, a patient will attend for a particular course of treatment (e.g., a number of restorative procedures) and then be absent for some time. Attendance rates and frequency tend to vary by both age and need. From experience, as with most areas of healthcare, female patients tend to attend more frequently, as a rule. With the demands of ageing, the older dentition often requires more attention, as older restorations require replacement. With this in mind, the longer-term relationship between dentist and patient becomes even more important. These can be challenging to manage – particularly with long absences between appointments/courses of treatment. The accurate, timely and contemporary recording of pertinent social history is a worthy tool to help support the dentist–patient relationship.

Relationships between the patient and other clinical team members should also not be overlooked. As dentistry is task-led, the dentist can often find themselves directly speaking with the patient for a limited amount of time. From the patient experience viewpoint, however, there can often be more interaction between patient and dental nurse and/or front desk staff.

Being mindful of these relationships and how they are fostered is of significant value to both service delivery and to the patient directly themselves. We know from the literature that the shared experience is often a key element of relationship skills. Being present with the patient at time of the procedure/check-up is often a building block for the care provider and the patient. The patient will often recall the nurse's name more readily than the dentist!

In thinking of relationships that are strictly outside the dental practice, the relationships we form with our specialist colleagues, medical practitioner colleagues, and laboratory technicians have significant value. The task-led nature of most dental procedures can (again) portray these interactions in a transactional light. However, with frequent contact, patient updates, clinical progress reports, and so on, the nature of these relationships need not just be solely transactional.

How to Foster Strong Relationships

Commonality plays a central role in relationship skills in clinical practice. This applies to both patient-dentist and dentist-team relationships. While the nature of dentistry as a service delivery profession is itself task-led, the relationships among the dental team should not be transactional or task-dependent. We know from the literature that shared experience and emphasizing our similarities assist in building fruitful, productive, and empowering relationships. It is easier to relate to people with whom we share a similarity. From a patient's perspective this can be as simple as a shared interest in sport, culture, or current affairs. From a team member's viewpoint this can be found routinely, in demonstrably showing the benefit of teamwork, career advancement, and value within the clinical working context. Providing this value for team members can take many forms. Ongoing clinical training and education are highly prized within a motivated and engaged team. Opportunities to advance in particular clinical interests (e.g., radiology, infection control, practice management, etc.) can provide a crucial support in fostering high-quality relationships too.

Further afield, the regular contact and communication with our specialist and allied healthcare colleagues is a good strategy. Due to the time-sensitive nature of most clinical needs in dentistry, we often find ourselves making contact in a time of patient need exclusively. A better strategy is contact when there is no need – and establishing a good dialogue founded on shared common goals. We each have our patients' interests at heart but contact outside of this clinical realm can be beneficial and supportive for both general practitioners and specialists. When was the last time you contacted your oral surgeon, endodontist, or periodontist and complimented them on a job well done for a patient you referred?

Examples of When Relationship Skills Worked Really Well/Went Wrong!

When employing a new dental nursing colleague, it's a smart strategy to encourage shadowing. The idea is simple. If you are to be part of our culture, it's smart to witness our culture in action. A day spent in the waiting room/surgery/sterilization room just observing the ebb and flow of patients and staff can yield a bounty of value. Often the relationships between staff, the camaraderie and shared goals of a clinic/team are clearly on view from these unscripted moments of a busy working day in a clinical environment.

An Example of Where a Relationship Worked Well

Employing a recently qualified dental nurse who has minimal previous dental surgery experience can provide an opportunity to create a long-lasting and high-quality relationship. The importance of culture can never be overstated. Drucker's famous line on "Culture eats strategy for breakfast" is a cardinal lesson to us all. By aligning the culture of your surgery with the needs of your staff, high-quality and enduring professional relationships can be forged. From the literature and experience, we all understand that relationships are best served from mutual benefit. Early and comprehensive induction can help foster shared goals, achievement, underline value, and create wins for all. One simple and novel method here is the practice telephone. Most practices rely on telephone as the first point of contact. Invariably, particularly in the morning, the telephone line can be busy. When a patient (whose relationship we value and continue to foster) telephones, it's often very encouraging to hear the practice message minder relate key details (name of practice, hours of opening, etc.). Added to this, it is often a good strategy to encourage each team member: dentist, nurse, manager, and so on to record the daily message minder script. This can help to underline commonality, reinforce purpose, shared goals, and help to further identify each member as a valued stakeholder.

An Example That Went Wrong

High-quality relationships thrive on commonality and shared experience. When a new staff member joins any team, it's often helpful to better understand their previous professional relationships and to demonstrate the culture in which they now find themselves. Though each individual clinical role within a dental team rarely differs, it is a very productive step to ensure that a full induction and expected responsibilities are highlighted and understood. This goes for all team members. Most practices encourage the custom of walking the patient from the waiting area to the surgery before treatment – and vice versa after treatment. The culture where I initially practiced mandated that the nurse undertakes this role. This can be instructive, as patients can tend to confide/discuss treatment with the nurse more than the dentist.

However, in another practice, it was mandated that the dentist walk the patient to the reception area after treatment. This was instilled to copper-fasten appointment setting. While both have inherent value, it needs to be crystal clear with the team which team member undertook the task. Relationships can suffer imbalance if one (or both) feel that all the initiative lies with one member only. By creating a space to allow contribution, it inherently conveys empowerment and not just simple delegation. It also means that, in the above case, the patient isn't left sitting waiting for someone to guide them to the surgery!

Conclusion

Healthcare relationships, and particularly those in dentistry, are often viewed from the dentist–patient viewpoint exclusively. While it is self-evident that the majority of time in any dental practice or clinic is spent in treatment, it is the relationships among the clinical team which deserve careful attention and nurturing. The individual members of a dental team represent the stakeholders of the practice. Developing high-quality relationships founded on equal status, common values (patient-centred care), shared experience (e.g., clinical training), and commonality make it easier to relate. Evidence of a highly functioning team filled with high-quality relationships promotes team well-being improves clinical outcomes and shines like a beacon to attending patients. Dentist–patient relationships thrive on the common sense of purpose (treatment outcome) and achievement of same. The synergistic nature of these relationships adds value and promotes clinical excellence.

References

Ha JF, Longnecker N. (2010). Doctor-patient communication: A review. *Ochsner J*, *10*(1), 38–43.
Lencioni PM. *The Five Dysfunctions of a Team*. Jossey-Bass; 2002.
Riess H. (2017). The science of empathy. *J Patient Exp*, *4*(2), 74–77.
Sherman JJ, Cramer A. (2005). Measurement of changes in empathy during dental school. *J Dent Educ*, *69*(3), 338–345.

7

EQ Critical Skill V

Self-Actualisation

MARY COLLINS

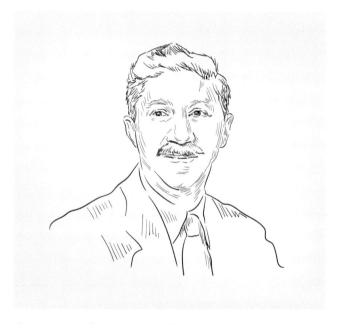

Introduction

Abraham Maslow, a key figure in humanistic psychology, provided many insights into the concept of self-actualisation. One of his notable quotes on this topic is:

> What a man can be, he must be. This needs we call self-actualisation…. It refers to the desire for self-fulfilment, namely, to the tendency for him to become actualised in what he is potentially. This tendency might be phrased as the desire to become more and more what one is, to become everything that one is capable of becoming.

This quote encapsulates Maslow's view on self-actualisation as a fundamental drive inherent in everyone, emphasising the importance of realising one's full potential and becoming the most that one can be.

This chapter will explore the following elements of self-actualisation as a critical skill for dentists at all career stages:

- A definition of self-actualisation
- Importance of this area in dentistry through all the career stages
- Practical ways to develop self-actualisation
- Dental practitioner perspective

Definition of Self-Actualisation

Self-actualisation is the state of achieving one's full potential and talents, which is seen as an inherent drive or need in every individual. The concept, often regarded as the epitome of psychological growth, was famously proposed by Abraham Maslow in the mid-20th century as the highest level in his hierarchy of needs.

In this seminal work, Maslow (1954) introduces and elaborates on the hierarchy of needs, culminating in self-actualisation as the ultimate psychological need. This book provides a comprehensive overview of his theory and its implications for psychology, education, and beyond, making it a foundational text for understanding human motivation and potential.

Maslow described self-actualisation as the desire to become more and more what one is, to become everything that one is capable of becoming. Individuals who achieve self-actualisation are characterised by a true understanding of their abilities, a deep sense of fulfilment, and the realisation of their potential. This is not a static state but a continuous process of becoming rather than a perfect state one reaches. It involves the growth of an individual beyond their normative needs, pursuing creative, meaningful activities, and peak experiences that contribute to a sense of wholeness and integration.

Self-actualised individuals tend to possess certain traits, including autonomy, authenticity, an appreciation for the simple things in life, deep relationships with a few rather than more superficial relationships with many, and a general sense of empathy and community feeling. They also exhibit problem-solving skills, creativity, and often have a democratic worldview.

It is important to note that Maslow later refined his model to include cognitive needs, aesthetic needs, and later, transcendence, as additional aspects that go beyond self-actualisation. Transcendence refers to the motivation to go beyond the personal self and to help others achieve self-actualisation.

Self-actualisation is a personal journey, unique in its expression and path for everyone. It represents the pursuit of reaching one's full potential, fostering an enduring commitment to growth and self-discovery.

In the context of the Emotional Capital Report (ECR) by RocheMartin, self-actualisation is defined as a key component of emotional intelligence that pertains to the pursuit and realisation of one's unique talents and capabilities. The ECR emphasises self-actualisation as critical for personal fulfilment and professional excellence, underlining its significance in contributing to one's sense of purpose and overall well-being.

Table 7.1   Self-Actualisation: Behaviours of High and Low Levels in the Workplace

HIGH SELF-ACTUALISATION BEHAVIOURS AT WORK	LOW SELF-ACTUALISATION BEHAVIOURS AT WORK
When someone possesses high levels of relationship skills, we see the following characteristics in their behaviour and interactions:	When someone possesses a low levels of relationship skills, we see the following characteristics in their behaviour and interactions:
1. *Innovative thinking*: They often approach problems with creative solutions and are not afraid to think outside the box.	1. *Lack of motivation*: They may seem disinterested or disengaged with their work, lacking passion or drive.
2. *Continuous learning*: Individuals are committed to personal and professional growth, actively seeking out new knowledge and skills.	2. *Fear of failure*: A tendency to avoid taking risks or pursuing challenging opportunities due to fear of failure or rejection.
3. *High levels of engagement*: Their work is characterised by enthusiasm and a deep sense of commitment, often going above and beyond what is required.	3. *Poor adaptability*: Struggle with change, finding it difficult to adjust to new situations or roles.
4. *Authenticity*: They are true to their values and beliefs, which is evident in their actions and decisions.	4. *Limited creativity*: They may stick to conventional approaches, showing reluctance to innovate or try new methods.
5. *Leadership*: High self-actualisers often inspire and motivate others, leading by example and fostering a positive team culture.	5. *Dependency*: Such individuals might overly rely on others for direction, lacking initiative or the ability to work independently.
6. *Resilience*: They exhibit the ability to bounce back from setbacks, viewing challenges as opportunities for growth.	6. *Unfulfilled potential*: Often, they do not reach their full professional potential, which can lead to feelings of dissatisfaction or frustration in the workplace.
7. *Goal-oriented*: Such individuals are focused on achieving their personal and professional goals, often setting high standards for themselves and others.	

Table 7.1 describes the behaviours we see in the workplace when Self-Actualisation is high and also when it is lacking.

High Levels of Self-Actualisation in the Workplace

Professionals who exhibit high levels of self-actualisation tend to demonstrate certain behaviours and attitudes that not only enhance their own career satisfaction but also contribute positively to their work environment:

- *Innovative thinking*: They often approach problems with creative solutions and are not afraid to think outside the box.
- *Continuous learning*: Individuals are committed to personal and professional growth, actively seeking out new knowledge and skills.
- *High levels of engagement*: Their work is characterised by enthusiasm and a deep sense of commitment, often going above and beyond what is required.
- *Authenticity*: They are true to their values and beliefs, which is evident in their actions and decisions.
- *Leadership*: High self-actualisers often inspire and motivate others, leading by example and fostering a positive team culture.
- *Resilience*: They exhibit the ability to bounce back from setbacks, viewing challenges as opportunities for growth.
- *Goal-oriented*: Such individuals are focused on achieving their personal and professional goals, often setting high standards for themselves and others.

Low Levels of Self-Actualisation in the Workplace

Conversely, professionals with low levels of self-actualisation may exhibit behaviours that could hinder their career development and negatively impact the workplace:

- *Lack of motivation*: They may seem disinterested or disengaged with their work, lacking passion or drive.
- *Fear of failure*: A tendency to avoid taking risks or pursuing challenging opportunities due to fear of failure or rejection.
- *Poor adaptability*: Struggle with change, finding it difficult to adjust to new situations or roles.
- *Limited creativity*: They may stick to conventional approaches, showing reluctance to innovate or try new methods.
- *Dependency*: Such individuals might overly rely on others for direction, lacking initiative or the ability to work independently.
- *Unfulfilled potential*: Often, they do not reach their full professional potential, which can lead to feelings of dissatisfaction or frustration in the workplace.

Why Is Self-Actualisation Important in Dentistry?

In the context of dentistry, the journey toward self-actualisation is a development path that influences practitioners from their student days to retirement. This continuous process of growth and development plays a pivotal role at every career stage, enhancing both personal satisfaction and professional excellence.

Dental Student

At the dental student phase, self-actualisation encompasses the mastery of technical skills and the cultivation of a professional identity grounded in empathy, integrity, and patient-centric values. Maslow (1954) describes this concept in "Motivation and Personality," suggesting that self-actualisation involves realising one's potential and striving for the highest form of personal development. For students, this means not only achieving academic and clinical competence but also developing a deep sense of professional purpose and ethics.

Early Career Dentist

As dentists transition into their early careers, they face the challenges of establishing themselves in clinical practice and forging meaningful professional relationships. Bandura's (1977) seminal theory of self-efficacy highlights the importance of belief in one's abilities as a foundation for achieving self-actualisation. For early career dentists, building confidence through continuous learning and practical experience is crucial. Engaging in professional development opportunities (e.g., mentorship) allows them to refine their skills and foster a positive identity as competent and compassionate care-givers. Developing meaningful relationships with patients and colleagues during this phase can significantly impact a dentist's ability to provide empathetic care, enhancing patient satisfaction and personal fulfilment in their work (Deci and Ryan, 2000).

Mid-Career Dentist

Mid-career dentists, often taking on leadership roles within their practices or the wider professional community, find self-actualisation in mentoring, community service, and professional advocacy. Dweck's (2006) concept of a growth mindset resonates with mid-career dentists' need for continual personal and professional growth. By embracing challenges, learning from failures, and contributing to the development of others, they fulfil their own potential while enriching the profession. This is also a phase when striking the right balance between personal and professional life is key to fulfilment.

Late Career Dentist

For dentists in the later stages of their careers, self-actualisation may focus on legacy, life reflection, and contributions beyond clinical practice. Viktor Frankl's (1959) "Man's Search for Meaning" emphasises the significance of finding purpose and fulfilment in life's endeavours. Late career dentists might pursue activities aligned with their deepest values, such as mentoring the next generation, engaging in volunteer work, or advocating for public health issues. These pursuits offer a sense of completion and satisfaction, marking the culmination of a lifelong journey toward self-actualisation. With people living and working longer, many people at the later part of their professional lives are now considering the "encore career." An encore career is a concept that refers to a new, often second, vocation that individuals pursue later in life, typically after retiring from their primary career. These careers are often characterised by a combination of continued income, personal meaning, and social impact, offering individuals an opportunity to align their work with their personal values and interests. Encore careers can be in various fields, including public service, education, healthcare, and the nonprofit sector. The term was popularised by Marc Freedman, founder of *Encore.org*, and emphasises the idea that individuals can pursue work that is both personally fulfilling and socially beneficial in the latter part of their lives.

The pursuit of self-actualisation in dentistry offers a framework for continuous personal and professional development. From the formative years of dental education to the reflective period of the late career, embracing the principles of self-actualisation fosters a fulfilling career. It enhances the quality of patient care, contributes to the dental community, and provides dentists with a profound sense of achievement and purpose.

How to Develop Self-Actualisation

Developing self-actualisation as a dentist involves embarking on a continuous journey of personal and professional growth aimed at realising one's full potential in both skills and character. Self-actualisation is the process of becoming the most that one can be; for dentists, this not only means achieving clinical excellence but also embodying the qualities of empathy, leadership, and lifelong learning. Below are practical strategies for dentists to develop self-actualisation, grounded in psychological theory and professional practice.

Embrace Lifelong Learning

- *Engage in continuous education*: Pursue advanced courses, certifications, and workshops beyond the required continuing dental education. This commitment to learning keeps you at the forefront of dental practices and technologies.
- *Develop knowledge beyond dentistry*: Explore subjects related to psychology, business management, or any area of personal interest. This broader knowledge base can enhance your understanding of patient care, practice management, and personal growth.

Cultivate Positive Emotional Intelligence Habits

- *Practice mindfulness*: Regular mindfulness practice can enhance self-awareness, a key component of emotional intelligence and self-actualisation. It helps in recognising one's emotional responses and managing them effectively in the workplace (Goleman, 2006).
- *Develop empathy*: Actively work to understand your patients' and colleagues' perspectives. This can improve patient satisfaction and staff relationships, fostering a positive practice environment that is more fulfilling for all.

Set Personal and Professional Goals

- *Define clear objectives*: Identify specific, measurable, achievable, relevant, and time-bound goals that align with your values and aspirations as a dentist (Locke and Latham, 2002).
- *Reflect regularly*: Make time for regular self-reflection on your goals, achievements, and areas for improvement. This reflective practice can guide your path to self-actualisation.

Seek Mentorship and Peer Support

- *Find a mentor*: Establish a mentorship relationship with a more experienced dentist who embodies the qualities you aspire to. This can provide guidance, inspiration, and practical advice on navigating the challenges of dental practice.

- *Engage in peer groups*: Join or form study groups, professional associations, or online communities with fellow dentists. Sharing experiences and challenges with peers can offer support and diverse perspectives on personal and professional growth.

Embrace Challenges and Setbacks

- *View failures as learning opportunities*: Adopt a growth mindset, viewing challenges and setbacks as opportunities to learn and grow. This resilience is key to pursuing self-actualisation despite the inevitable difficulties encountered in practice (Dweck, 2006).
- *Take calculated risks*: Step out of your comfort zone by taking on new challenges, whether it's learning a new dental technique, opening a practice, or leading a professional organisation. These experiences can stimulate personal and professional growth.

Practice Self-Care and Well-Being

- *Prioritise physical health*: Regular exercise, a balanced diet, and adequate rest are fundamental for maintaining the physical stamina required for demanding dental procedures.
- *Maintain positive mental health*: Engage in activities that promote mental well-being, such as hobbies, socialising, or therapy. Balancing the stresses of dental practice with personal well-being is crucial for sustained self-actualisation.

Contribute to the Community

- *Volunteer and advocacy*: Participate in community outreach programmes, provide free dental care to underserved populations, or advocate for public health policies. Contributing to the well-being of the community can fulfil a sense of purpose and advance one's journey towards self-actualisation.
- *Mentor future dentists*: Share your knowledge and experience by mentoring dental students or young dentists. This not only contributes to the profession but also enriches your sense of accomplishment and growth.

Conclusion

Developing self-actualisation as a dentist requires a multifaceted approach that encompasses lifelong learning, emotional intelligence, goal setting, mentorship, resilience, self-care, and community service. By embracing these strategies, dentists can not only achieve professional excellence but also realise their fullest potential as compassionate caregivers, effective leaders, and fulfilled individuals. The journey to self-actualisation is both personal and professional, offering a path to a rewarding career and a meaningful career in dentistry.

SELF-ACTUALISATION: DENTAL PRACTITIONER PERSPECTIVE

IAN WILSON

Self-actualisation – A concept introduced by Abraham Maslow: "What a man can be, he must be. This need we call self-actualisation" – is about reaching our full potential and embracing our talents and capabilities, representing the pinnacle of emotional and psychological growth.

In the realm of dentistry, the journey towards self-actualisation significantly shapes dental clinicians' personal growth and professional journey. It deeply influences how they engage with their work, connect with patients, and find satisfaction in their careers. Dental professionals growing in this emotional intelligence competency are able to maintain an enthusiastic commitment to long-term goals, achieving a level of work–life balance and satisfaction from their accomplishments.

Developing self-actualisation as an emotional competency is the real source of power behind sustained high performance. The skilful development and management of your emotional energy will ultimately determine the quality of your productivity at work and in life generally (Newman, 2008; Newman and Purse, 2007).

Let's explore the emotional intelligence perspective on the impact of varying degrees of self-actualisation for a dental clinician (Wason, 2023).

High Self-Actualisation

1. *Empathetic patient care*: Dentists embracing their full potential are more passionate and driven to excel in patient care. They continuously hone their skills and stay abreast of dental innovations, leading to a compassionate and comprehensive approach to treating patients. How will we understand that empathy involves the components of active listening, curiosity in the patient in front of you and that emotional attachment, then a passionate clinician will by nature and by habit become a much more empathic commission to their patients?

2. *Fulfilling career experience*: Achieving self-actualisation brings a profound sense of fulfilment and contentment in one's career. For dental professionals, this translates into taking pride in their work, which not only mitigates burnout but also enhances their overall well-being. Where a clinician has the motivation and the self-awareness to recognise that the more energy and resources they put into their own self-development (skills and knowledge) then the more satisfying and fulfilling their clinical career and their leadership within the profession will be.

3. *Creative leadership*: Dentists who have reached a high level of self-actualisation often lead by example, showing creativity in their work and inspiring those

DOI: 10.1201/9781003379829-13

around them. They contribute to dental advancements, engage in research, and mentor emerging talents in the field.

4. *Whole-person care approach*: A self-actualised dentist sees beyond the teeth, considering the overall health and well-being of their patients. This holistic perspective fosters a more comprehensive and empathetic approach to patient care, leading to superior health outcomes. A clinician who understands the importance of self-actualisation has reached that place in their professional career where they are naturally able to perform in the flow state (Csikszentmihalyi, 1990; see also Moore, 2019) that fuels their passion.

Tasks within dentistry that foster a state of flow often exhibit similar traits. These tasks are typically:

- Appropriately challenging, providing a sense of difficulty without being overwhelming.
- Intrinsically rewarding, offering satisfaction or purpose to the individual engaging in them.
- Substantial, requiring a genuine investment of time and effort to progress.

Indications that someone is in a state of flow include:

- Unwavering focus, making it difficult for external distractions to disrupt their engagement in the task.
- Reduced self-awareness, with a decline in self-centred thoughts or concerns about performance and perception by others.
- Genuine enjoyment of the activity, prompting deep immersion and absorption in the experience.
- Willingness to persist even in the face of challenges, as flow can help mitigate frustration and enable the continued pursuit of goals.

Low Self-Actualisation

1. *Stunted professional development*: Dental clinicians struggling to reach self-actualisation may find themselves in a professional rut, less inclined to pursue new knowledge or adopt innovative practices, which can hamper their effectiveness and growth. The motivation to take risks is stunted!

2. *Career dissatisfaction and burnout*: Lacking the drive for personal and professional growth can leave dentists feeling unfulfilled, contributing to increased feelings of burnout, dissatisfaction, and potentially, depression.

3. *Compromised patient care*: Without the motivation for self-improvement, the quality of care provided to patients may decline. Such clinicians might not be as thorough or as engaged with their patients, affecting patient satisfaction and outcomes.

4. *Limited contributions to dentistry*: A dentist not striving for self-actualisation may contribute less in terms of innovation, research, and leadership within the field, impacting not only their career path but also the progression of their dental practice.

Within emotional intelligence, self-actualisation is made up of two main emotional components: passion and a work–life balance that facilitates setting creative goals.

Passion

Having a passion for what you do is crucial. It empowers you to inspire and lead others, starting each day with enthusiasm for your work and excitement to collaborate with your team and care for your patients. To fuel your passion, pay attention to what invigorates you and what you find engaging. For example, I vividly recall feeling passionate when I first stepped into a clinic in Sub-Saharan Africa, realising how my professional skills could positively impact those in need.

To achieve self-actualisation, it's essential to ensure that your skills match the challenges you face, set clear goals, focus on developing leadership qualities, take control of your growth, maintain a positive attitude, learn from each experience, avoid seeking constant admiration, and embrace self-awareness and feedback.

Passionate individuals are productive, persistent high performers who seek creative challenges, enjoy learning, and take pride in their work. They thrive on improvement and exhibit unwavering energy for discovering new possibilities.

Work–Life Balance

The second aspect of self-actualisation involves creating a balance between work and personal life. By setting goals, following a plan, and taking action in response to creative challenges, you can enhance your emotional well-being and ensure that all important aspects of your life receive adequate attention. It is crucial to avoid being solely consumed by work or any specific task, such as providing dental care, as neglecting other areas can have a significant impact on your long-term happiness. I have observed situations where colleagues have experienced this imbalance, resulting in emotional exhaustion and a toll on their relationships with loved ones.

Embracing emotional intelligence in dentistry underscores the importance of self-actualisation in enhancing a clinician's connection with their work and patients, as well as their personal job satisfaction. Fostering a culture within the workplace that values continuous learning, emotional growth, and professional development can empower dental professionals to achieve higher levels of self-actualisation, enriching their careers, their teams, and the quality of care they provide.

Case Study 1

Chris a young foundation dentist came to see me for some coaching because he was concerned that he had got into a rut of dissatisfaction during his training year. He felt that he was just doing the bare minimum to tick the box and wasn't achieving any sense of purpose at this early stage of his career.

As we explored this emotional competency, we discovered that the discontent for him lay with a negative experience as an undergraduate but this had coloured the value that he placed upon himself and the contribution that he felt he could make to the profession.

We spent some time exploring valuing who he was that he made a massive difference to the patients he was treating on a day-to-day basis and that he was in a unique opportunity during his training year to develop the skills significantly. We looked at his patient satisfaction questionnaires where the feedback was outstanding but the negative narrative he had "agreed" with had eroded his initial passion and drive for professional excellence.

Once we had identified this, Chris was then able to recognise that he was empowered to set some more challenging goals for his training year and subsequently the increased energy and focus for his training allowed him to take more risks. Thus, achieving greater job satisfaction in the workplace. This new energy and drive not only had a direct consequence for his training outcomes but gave him a vision of his professional career next steps.

Case Study 2

Anisha was a 45-year-old dental practice owner, married to her husband for 20 years with two young children. Due to the pressures of running her busy mixed practice, she found herself coming home exhausted, bringing her stresses of the workplace into her home and not being able to switch off. This resulted in a degree of conflict with her husband, and she was frustrated with her inability to leave the issues of work there and spend quality time with her family when she got home. She also felt that she had lost her clear purpose and direction. Work had become "all consuming."

We used a simple audit tool for looking at the seven key areas of life (Boldt, 2004) that are important for all of us:

- Social and family relationships
- Career and educational aspirations
- Financial security
- Physical health/leisure
- Life's routine responsibilities
- Society and contribution
- Mental, emotional, and inner well-being

We were, therefore, able to identify where she was currently prioritising and where she needed instead to focus to result in a more meaningful work-life balance so that the important areas in her life got the time and energy they deserve. Being able to agree with those closest to her in this reprioritising resulted in new energy for the practice and leaving the natural day-to-day stresses of work where they belonged – at work! In her personal life, she was able to identify where time with her husband and children gave her the energy and passion, she needed to continue her professional career and ongoing development of her skills.

Tips for Developing Your Self-Actualisation

- *Improving professional development*: Dentists who value personal growth know how important it is to keep learning. They're always keen to try new techniques, use the latest technology, and stay up to date with the newest research. This dedication ensures they provide top-quality care and helps them grow both personally and professionally. Striving for excellence not only enhances their practice but also gives them a real sense of achievement in helping people look after their oral health.
- *Growing personally*: For dentists aiming for self-improvement, personal development is key. Balancing work and personal interests are essential for staying mentally healthy and avoiding burnout. By finding a mix of professional responsibilities and personal hobbies, dentists can boost their mental well-being, job satisfaction, and overall happiness.
- *Giving back*: Self-improving dentists understand the importance of giving back to their communities. They don't just focus on personal growth but also give back through volunteering, mentoring, and educational projects, making a lasting impact beyond their clinic.
- *Workplace environment*: Creating a positive workplace relies on encouraging personal growth. Dentists who have achieved personal growth play a crucial role in building a work culture where teamwork, support, open communication, respect, and professional development are promoted among colleagues. This kind of atmosphere not only boosts job satisfaction but also benefits the dentist's overall well-being.

Finally!

The process of self-actualisation is about becoming all that you can be and doing all that you can do. It will enable others to believe they can do the same.

The path to being a top-notch dentist is all about balancing your professional skills with personal development and making a positive impact on the world. By staying motivated, building strong professional and personal connections, always learning, finding time for yourself, and giving back, dentists can truly change their lives and careers for the better. This approach doesn't just bring more satisfaction, it also improves patient care and outcomes, making the dental industry as a whole better.

References

Bandura AJ (1977). *Social Learning Theory*. Prentice Hall.

Boldt LG (2004). *How to Find the Work You Love*. Penguin.

Csikszentmihalyi M (1990). *Flow: The Psychology of Optimal Experience*. Harper & Row.

Deci EL, Ryan RM (2000). The "what" and "why" of goal pursuits: Human needs and the self-determination of behavior. *Psychological Inquiry*, *11*(4), 227.

Dweck CS (2006). *Mindset: The New Psychology of Success*. Random House.

Frankl V (1959). *Man's Search for Meaning*. Beacon Press.

Goleman D (2006). *Social Intelligence: The New Science of Human Relationships*. Bantam Books.

Locke EA, Latham GP (2002). Building a practically useful theory of goal setting and task motivation: A 35-year odyssey. *American Psychologist*, *57*(9), 705–717.

Maslow AH (1954). Motivation and Personality. Harper & Row.

Moore C (2019) What Is Flow in Positive Psychology? (Incl. 10+ Activities) [internet]. *Positive Psychology*. Available at: https://positivepsychology.com/what-is-flow/

Newman M (2008). *Emotional Capitalists: The New Leaders – Building Emotional Intelligence and Leadership Success*. Wiley.

Newman M, Purse J (2007). *Technical Manual – The Emotional Capital Report*. RocheMartin Pty Ltd.

Wason R (2023). The self-actualised dentist. *J Dent Mat*, *1*(1), 31–33.

8

MOVING FORWARD

Developing Your EQ over a Lifetime

MARY COLLINS

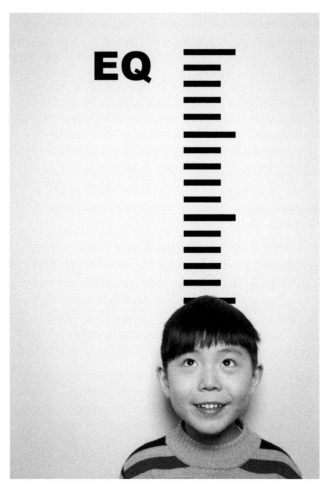

(*Source*: https://www.gettyimages.co.uk/detail/photo/boy-measuring-emotional-intelligence-royalty-free-image/170024553?adppopup=true)

Introduction

This final chapter focuses on the continuous journey of emotional and professional development in dentistry. This chapter explores the significance of emotional intelligence (EQ) in shaping both interpersonal interactions and personal career progression. Key topics covered include:

DOI: 10.1201/9781003379829-14

- *Neuroplasticity*: The brain's remarkable ability to form new neural connections, allowing for the adoption of new behaviours and attitudes. This section emphasises the scientific underpinning of behavioural change and its relevance to EQ development.
- *Key success factors for positive change*: Identification and exploration of critical elements that facilitate meaningful personal and professional transformation, highlighting the importance of resilience and empathy in the dental profession.
- *EQ self-assessment and development plan*: A step-by-step guide for evaluating one's emotional competencies, creating a strategic plan for growth. This process serves as a foundation for recognising emotional strengths and pinpointing areas for improvement.
- *10 tips to stay on track*: Practical recommendations designed to sustain focus and motivation on the path to emotional development. These tips provide actionable strategies to ensure continued progress and fulfilment.
- *Practitioner perspective*: Role of coaching in dentistry: Examination of the important support system coaching offers within the dental field.

This chapter is designed to offer comprehensive insights and strategies for cultivating EQ across the professional lifespan of a dentist. Whether at the beginning stages of one's dental career or amidst the complexities of an established practice, this chapter presents a blueprint for developing EQ as a means to enhance both personal well-being and the quality of patient care.

Rewiring Your Brain to Develop New Behaviours

Neuroplasticity, or the brain's capacity to form new neural pathways, fundamentally underpins our ability to adapt, learn, and modify our behaviour and attitudes throughout life. This dynamic quality of the brain is critical in the context of developing emotional intelligence (EQ) and is particularly relevant in professions requiring high levels of interpersonal interaction and stress management, such as dentistry.

In dentistry, the application of neuroplasticity extends beyond clinical skills and technical knowledge to encompass emotional and psychological adaptability. The ability to manage one's emotions, understand those of others, and adapt to the continuously evolving landscape of dental practice is invaluable. As Doidge (2007) posits in *The Brain That Changes Itself* the realisation that the brain is not fixed but rather malleable opens up vast possibilities for personal and professional growth.

Neuroplasticity provides a scientific foundation for the development of new behaviours and attitudes necessary for effective dental practice. This includes enhancing communication skills, developing empathy, and managing stress and anxiety – both one's own and that of the patients. Research by Davidson and McEwen (2012) demonstrates that sustained practices, such as mindfulness and stress reduction techniques, can lead to structural changes in the brain associated with increased emotional regulation and resilience. For dentists, this means that actively engaging in practices designed to enhance EQ can lead to tangible changes in the brain, thereby improving their capacity to connect with patients, manage challenging situations, and maintain personal well-being.

The adoption of new behaviours and attitudes is a critical aspect of continuous professional development in dentistry. Whether it is adopting new clinical techniques, integrating new technologies into practice, or enhancing patient communication, the ability to learn and adapt is essential. The principles of neuroplasticity suggest that with repeated practice and exposure, dentists can train their brains to become more efficient and effective in these areas. This is supported by the work of Merzenich (2013) who highlights the role of repetitive practice in strengthening neural connections and facilitating skill acquisition.

Emotional intelligence, which encompasses self-awareness, self-regulation, motivation, empathy, and social skills, is increasingly recognised as a cornerstone of successful dental practice. The development of EQ is a lifelong process that can be significantly enhanced by understanding and leveraging neuroplasticity. For instance, practices such as reflective listening, empathy training, and emotional regulation exercises can, over time, lead to changes in brain regions associated with emotional intelligence (Goleman, 1995). This not only improves interactions with patients and colleagues but also contributes to a more fulfilling personal and professional life overall.

Below are three practical ways to support neuroplasticity for dentists:

- *Mindfulness and meditation*: Regular mindfulness practice can enhance concentration, emotional regulation, and empathy, crucial components of EQ in dentistry. This is due to the impact of mindfulness on the brain's structure and function, particularly in areas related to attention and emotion regulation (Hölzel et al., 2011).
- *Emotional regulation training*: Techniques designed to manage stress, such as deep breathing, cognitive reframing, and relaxation exercises, can help dentists navigate the high-pressure environment of dental practice, reducing burnout and improving patient care.
- *Continued learning and skill development*: Engaging in ongoing professional development and learning new skills can stimulate neuroplasticity, keeping the brain agile and ensuring dentists remain at the forefront of their field.

The concept of neuroplasticity offers an exciting framework for understanding and facilitating behavioural change and EQ development in dentistry. By recognising that the brain is capable of remarkable adaptation and growth, dental professionals can harness this potential to enhance their practice, improve patient care, and achieve personal and professional fulfilment. Through targeted strategies and sustained effort, dentists can reshape their neural pathways, leading to lasting improvements in emotional intelligence and overall well-being.

Key Success Factors for Positive Change

Developing your EQ is not just about practising specific techniques; it also requires an understanding of the key factors that contribute to successful emotional growth.

1. **Consistency and Patience**

   The development of emotional intelligence is dependent on regular, consistent practice. Like a muscle that strengthen and grows through continuous exercise, EQ develops with the persistent application of skills such as emotional awareness, empathy, and self-regulation. Integrating EQ practices into daily routines ensures the gradual transformation of these skills from conscious efforts to subconscious habits. In his best-selling book *Atomic Habits*, James Clear emphasises the significance of small changes and consistency with the insight: "Success is the product of daily habits – not once-in-a-lifetime transformations" (Clear, 2018). This quote demonstrates the importance of the cumulative effect of small, consistent actions over grand, isolated efforts in achieving lasting behavioural change and success.

   Enhancing one's EQ is a process that unfolds over time, necessitating patience. Significant emotional growth, particularly in altering deep-seated habits and responses, does not occur instantly. Patience allows for a kinder, more forgiving approach to personal development, acknowledging that progress often comes in increments. Psychologist Daniel Goleman (1995) discusses the importance of patience in emotional learning, highlighting that understanding and changing emotional responses is a gradual journey that requires time and dedication.

2. **Openness to Feedback**

   Feedback from others is invaluable for identifying blind spots in our emotional behaviours and areas for improvement. Being open to receiving constructive feedback – and actively seeking it – can accelerate EQ development. This concept is supported by David R. Caruso and Peter Salovey who highlight the importance of feedback for leaders seeking to develop emotional intelligence in their work. "Feedback is the breakfast of champions, and it is especially nutritious when you are growing your emotional intelligence. Leaders need to know how their emotions and actions affect others, and feedback provides this critical insight" (Caruso and Salovey, 2004).

3. **Self-Compassion**

   The path to enhance emotional quotient (EQ) is undeniably fraught with obstacles and setbacks over a dentist's lifetime. The cultivation of self-compassion emerges as a pivotal factor in sustaining and nurturing their emotional growth and development. Self-compassion, characterised by an empathetic and understanding approach towards oneself during times of failure or difficulty, serves as a critical tool in the development of EQ. This practice is not merely an exercise in self-indulgence but a strategic approach to fostering a resilient and adaptive leadership style.

In her seminal study from 2003, Kristin Neff outlined the enormous impact that self-compassion has on personal growth. She highlighted the power of self-compassion to foster resilience, inspire persistence, and reduce the demoralising impacts of setbacks and failures.

For dentists, this implies that integrating self-compassion into their developmental toolkit can significantly enhance their ability to weather the inherent challenges of EQ growth.

Self-compassion facilitates a nurturing environment for emotional intelligence to flourish by allowing professionals to acknowledge their vulnerabilities and limitations without harsh judgement. This acceptance enables them to view mistakes not as insurmountable barriers to their leadership efficacy but as invaluable learning opportunities. It shifts the focus from a punitive perspective of self-critique to a constructive one, fostering an atmosphere where growth is nurtured through understanding and kindness.

In addition to bolstering resilience, self-compassion has been shown to enhance motivation. Contrary to the belief that self-compassion might lead to complacency, Neff's research suggests that individuals who practice self-compassion are more likely to embrace personal growth and improvement. For leaders, this means that self-compassion can serve as a motivator for continuous EQ development, inspiring them to set and pursue ambitious emotional intelligence goals with persistence and dedication.

Furthermore, self-compassion equips leaders with the emotional bandwidth to extend the same level of understanding and empathy to others. This outward projection of compassion can significantly improve interpersonal relationships, conflict resolution, and team dynamics, key components of effective leadership. By modelling self-compassion, leaders can inspire their teams to adopt a similar stance, fostering an environment where emotional support and personal development are valued.

Embracing these core principles – consistency and patience, openness to feedback, and self-compassion – equips individuals with the mindset and practices necessary for developing high levels of EQ. This comprehensive approach not only fosters personal and professional fulfilment but also lays the groundwork for a lifetime of emotional growth and learning.

EQ Self-Assessment and Development Plan

To effectively develop your EQ, it's crucial to start with a self-assessment to understand your current emotional intelligence level. Measuring EQ provides a baseline from which individuals can identify strengths and pinpoint areas for improvement. Understanding one's emotional competencies facilitates targeted personal development efforts, enabling individuals to focus on enhancing specific skills that can lead to more effective communication, better relationship management, and improved problem-solving abilities.

For leaders, EQ is a critical determinant of their ability to inspire, motivate, and connect with their teams. An accurate assessment of a leader's EQ can highlight essential insights into their leadership style, including their capacity for empathy, adaptability, and resilience. These insights enable leaders to refine their approach, fostering a positive work environment and driving team performance.

In organisational settings, measuring the EQ of team members can illuminate the dynamics that influence team interactions and performance. Understanding the emotional strengths and vulnerabilities within a team allows for the strategic allocation of roles and responsibilities, enhancing collaboration and minimising conflict.

Beyond individual and team levels, assessing EQ across an organisation can guide strategic development initiatives. It identifies cultural strengths and areas requiring attention, informing training programs, and interventions that cultivate a supportive and emotionally intelligent organisational culture.

The RocheMartin Emotional Capital Report (ECR)

The RocheMartin ECR stands out as a sophisticated tool for assessing emotional intelligence. Developed through rigorous research and grounded in psychological theory, the ECR offers a comprehensive evaluation of the key dimensions of emotional intelligence that are critical for effective leadership and professional success. The tool provides detailed insights into an individual's emotional strengths and potential areas for development, making it an invaluable resource for personal growth and leadership enhancement.

The ECR is supported by empirical research, ensuring that its assessments are both reliable and valid. This evidence-based foundation assures users that the insights gained from the ECR are grounded in solid psychological principles, providing a trustworthy basis for development efforts.

While the ECR is applicable across various contexts, its focus on leadership competencies makes it particularly useful for individuals in or aspiring to leadership roles. The tool assesses emotional skills essential for leadership, such as emotional self-awareness, empathy, adaptability, and influence, providing leaders with targeted feedback that can inform their personal and professional development strategies.

Beyond merely assessing EQ, the ECR offers actionable insights and recommendations for development. This feature makes it an effective instrument not just for measurement but also for facilitating growth. Individuals can leverage the ECR's feedback to craft personalised development plans that enhance their emotional intelligence over time.

In conclusion, measuring emotional intelligence is a critical step for individuals aiming to enhance their professional effectiveness, leadership capabilities, and personal well-being. The RocheMartin ECR offers a scientifically grounded, comprehensive tool for assessing and developing the emotional competencies that underpin success across various domains. By providing detailed, actionable insights into one's

EQ, the ECR serves as an essential resource for anyone committed to achieving personal growth and professional excellence.

Based on the assessment results, create a personalised development plan that targets your specific needs. This plan should include specific, measurable, achievable, relevant, and time-bound (SMART) goals, along with strategies for achieving them.

10 Tips to Stay on Track

1. *Set clear goals*: Define what you want to achieve in your EQ development journey and why it's important to you.
2. *Practice active listening*: Improve your social skills by listening actively to others, showing empathy, and understanding their perspectives.
3. *Keep a journal*: Reflect on your daily emotional experiences and reactions to enhance self-awareness.
4. *Seek new experiences*: Expose yourself to new situations and people to broaden your emotional and social skills.
5. *Learn to manage stress*: Develop healthy coping mechanisms for stress, such as exercise, relaxation techniques, or hobbies.
6. *Cultivate positivity*: Focus on positive emotions and gratitude to enhance your mood and outlook. End each day with a gratitude practice – e.g., three good things, which simply involves reflecting on three positive things that happened to you that day that you are grateful for.
7. *Improve your non-verbal communication*: Be mindful of your body language, facial expressions, and tone of voice as they play a key role in effective communication.
8. *Work with a mentor*: Work with a mentor to develop your leadership capability, select a mentor with strengths in the areas you want to develop in.
9. *Embrace empathy*: Try to see situations from others' points of view and respond with understanding and compassion.
10. *Stay curious and open-minded*: Maintain a "growth mindset" willingness to learn and grow, both emotionally and intellectually.

Conclusion

Developing your emotional intelligence is a lifelong journey that requires dedication, practice, and a commitment to continuous growth. By rewiring your brain to develop new behaviours, identifying key success factors, conducting EQ self-assessments, and implementing practical tips to stay on track, you can enhance your emotional intelligence and enjoy the myriad benefits it brings to your personal and professional life. Remember, the pursuit of emotional intelligence is not just about personal achievement; it's about enriching your relationships, improving your well-being, and contributing positively to the world around you. Embrace this journey with an open heart and mind and watch as your life transforms in the most remarkable ways.

DENTAL PRACTITIONER PERSPECTIVE: COACHING IN DENTISTRY

RORY O'REILLY

Introduction

The aim of this piece is to introduce coaching to the reader and consider its potential benefits for dental practitioners developing their emotional intelligence. Being a relatively novel subject in dentistry, the discussion will integrate seminal and contemporary literature from both healthcare and coaching contexts and be grounded in everyday examples from dental practice. The section will conclude with a practical guide to effective engagement with coaching as a dental practitioner.

What Is Coaching?

Coaching is a fundamentally heterogeneous field of practice, owing to its eclectic origin story and the diversity of contributing areas of knowledge. While the literature is replete with definitions, as one might expect, absolute uniformity is lacking. To avoid further complicating the definitional landscape, the author refers to a recent, robust definition proposed by Cox et al. (2023, p. 2):

> Coaching is a human development process that involves structured, focused interaction and the use of appropriate strategies, tools and techniques to promote desirable and sustainable change for the benefit of the client and potentially for other stakeholders.

This can be characterised further by considering the components of some archetypal coaching scenarios. Coaching is classically an interpersonal process; the interaction is between a coach and client (or "coachee"). It is conversational and, while often dyadic, may involve a coach engaging larger groups. The strategies and techniques that guide these conversations stem from an expanding range of contributing theories including various traditions of psychology (including psychodynamic, humanistic, cognitive-behavioural, developmental, transpersonal, and positive psychology), management science, adult learning theory, neuroscience, and philosophy (Boyatzis and Jack, 2018; Cox et al., 2023). The context of a given conversation, client preferences, the coach's background, and their experience typically dictate the specific methods applied. While coaching typically implies a series of conversations, the number and duration vary. This is reflected plainly in the literature with study designs implementing single sessions of 30 minutes up to eight sessions of one hour (Boet et al., 2023). What remains central in any coaching engagement is the intended change. This is the anticipated

DOI: 10.1201/9781003379829-15

endpoint, irrespective of whether a single or a dozen sessions are expected. It is established explicitly at the beginning of any coaching process and is self-determined by the coachee. Occasionally, it may be decided in collaboration with other stakeholders like line managers in a corporate environment. While coaching in the context of business is becoming increasingly popular, it has also been implemented in education, sport, healthcare, and personal settings among others (Boet et al., 2023; International Coaching Federation, 2023; van Niewerburgh, 2012; Whitmore, 2009).

In developing a well-rounded understanding of coaching, it is important to distinguish it from some of its close relatives; namely mentoring, consulting, psychotherapy, training, and instruction. Indeed, this is one of the main challenges in creating a definition that is adequately precise. While these are discrete areas of practice, certain parallels exist and at times they can overlap. Training and instruction can be recognised by a prescriptive position of the trainer or instructor. They prescribe a course of action to their clients. Conversely, coaches tend to hold a non-directive stance and avoid the assumption that "they know best." The coach's role is to assist the coachee in unpicking his situation to understand his best course of action. Mentoring and consulting imply that the service provider has an expert knowledge or first-hand experience of the subject matter that the client presents. In coaching, this is not necessarily the case. A coach aims to bring structure to the client's thinking in pursuit of clarity and progress. This does not require, or indeed preclude a coach from holding specific knowledge on the topic. Psychotherapy commonly addresses mental health diagnoses in clinical populations. This is not the remit of a coach. Psychotherapy considers troubling events from a client's past, having a more retrospective focus, whereas coaching is more proactive and prospective, or future focused. However, contemporary literature considers mental health to exist on a spectrum; the boundary between health and ill-health, clinical and non-clinical issues is indistinct (Khwaja, 2023). It's critical to appreciate that the hallmarks of these related fields are not exclusive. At times, coaches may adopt a more prescriptive or directive position, hold expert knowledge on the subject matter, or engage with client's who are struggling with mental health concerns. You can see how drawing firm lines between them is difficult. A dental analogy may illustrate this point further.

Within dentistry, there are several subspecialties: oral surgery, periodontics, endodontics, and orthodontics among others. Although these specialties are discrete areas of practice, none of them exist in isolation from the other. In certain circumstances, they overlap. Consider the practice of a specialist periodontist. Invariably, they will encounter necrotic pulps and occlusal interferences that will present with associated disturbances in the periodontium. The periodontist must acknowledge the limits of their scope of practice, understand related specialties, take account of the patient's wishes and the desired endpoint, and be willing to refer where appropriate. This is analogous to how a coach engages with a coachee. Perhaps coaching in isolation is the best course of action. Perhaps adjunctive measures from a related field are needed in tandem. Perhaps a referral to a different service entirely is warranted.

A final consideration to fully grasp the concept of coaching involves discerning between coaching as a practice and coaching as an approach or philosophy. What has been described thus far is coaching as a practice – the structured interaction of a coach with an individual or group of coachees. The term coaching is also used to describe a style of approach – a set of skills and values that would typically be found in a coaching conversation but have been adapted to a broader context. These might include listening, empathy, honesty, respect, and autonomy. Coaching leadership is a useful example. It describes the way in which a leader relates to and supports their organisation and team members. While it absolutely may involve the specific practice of coaching, it also refers to the priorities and focus of the leader (Hwang et al., 2023).

Coaching and Dentistry

Coaching first appeared in the dental literature in the late 1980s. At that time, publications on the subject were infrequent. Most originated from the United States and focused on themes related to practice management, dental education, and behaviour management in paediatric patients (Adams, 1988; Metzger Samuels, 1991; Pinkham, 1993). More recently, interest in the applications of coaching in dentistry has burgeoned. While the topics of dental education and behaviour management remain present, other areas like leadership in dentistry, clinician well-being, and patient-centred care have also been explored through the lens of coaching. With research contributions emerging across the globe, the volume and frequency of publication has seen a marked uptick in the last five years (Aboalshamat et al., 2020; Maragha et al., 2023; Plessas et al., 2022; Stormon et al., 2022). This trend mirrors a bolstered interest in the social sciences more generally, which has assumed a more prominent position in contemporary healthcare literature (Chai et al., 2021; Murariu et al., 2019; Willumsen et al., 2022).

What Are the Benefits?

Before examining the specific benefits of coaching in dentistry, a brief look at coaching outcomes more broadly is warranted given the longer history of writing on the subject. Athanasopoulou and Dopson's (2018) systematic review highlights a diverse range of outcomes in a corporate setting. Coaching was found to positively affect the client on both a personal and professional level. Coachees improved resilience, goal setting, and time management, while experiencing reduced stress and anxiety. They developed better communication, management, and leadership skills, and felt more valued at work. Indirect effects related to organisation productivity and culture also featured. The applicability of these findings to healthcare workers and their institutions is obvious and likely contributed to the currently expanding research interest.

In dentistry, coaching has the potential to enhance various dimensions of our personal and professional development, many of which map neatly onto the critical skills of the emotional capital framework. Distinguishing between personal and professional growth serves as a useful schema.

Professional Development

In the author's experience of coaching and dentistry, there are three central areas of benefit to be considered:

- Technical aspects of clinical dentistry
- How we care for our patients
- How we engage with our colleagues

Dentistry is a uniquely challenging occupation that invariably involves clinical complications and failures. Our attitudes to this reality of dental practice are pivotal in determining its impact. The work of Carol Dweck (2017) on growth and fixed mindsets has made this patently clear. Consider the example of a newly qualified dentist working in general practice. They take on a challenging root canal treatment on an upper first molar that goes awry. A file fractures, the patient is duly dissatisfied, and the dentist leaves work disheartened. A growth mindset in this scenario would be characterised by a curiosity in what went wrong, efforts to improve, and a continued willingness to engage with appropriate levels of challenge. A fixed mindset, however, would be associated with future avoidance of similar challenges, and maladaptive beliefs that undermine strategies to learn and improve, ultimately stalling or even eroding our clinical skills. Many coaches are well-versed in cognitive behavioural techniques useful in addressing unhelpful beliefs and attitudes that hold us back. This approach, combined with coaching's established ability to improve client goal setting, could help dental practitioners deal with inevitable failures and sustain a commitment to clinical progression (Burt and Talati, 2017; Grant and Atad, 2022; Theeboom et al., 2014).

However, practising dentistry goes beyond hard skills and technical proficiencies. Contemporary healthcare has embraced patient-centred care, a departure from traditional biomedical models which were "paternalistic, provider-driven and disease-focused" (Fix et al., 2018, p. 301). Patient-centred care emphasises an appreciation of the patient's "biography," the impact of their condition and their attitudes to it (Mead and Bower, 2000, p. 1088). It advocates for shared decision-making and stresses the importance of the patient-doctor relationship. These elements imply advanced communication skills, a robust capacity to listen, and genuine empathy. To truly deliver patient-centred care with consistency is difficult. It requires practice and commitment. It takes more time and certainly asks more of us as clinicians. However, it has been associated with improved health outcomes and patient satisfaction (Fix et al., 2018). All the tenets of patient-centred care are typical of a coaching relationship. In a qualitative study of American medical physicians, receiving coaching, and experiencing these interpersonal mechanics first-hand, translated to improvements in patient care. Physicians reported a renewed awareness of the importance of these elements of their role and an increased capacity to implement them (Schneider et al., 2014). It is the author's view that they are particularly valuable when managing conflict or handling difficult patient emotions. Indeed, the management of dental phobia has integrated many overlapping concepts from cognitive behavioural psychology (Hauge et al., 2022).

Another useful application of coaching in how we care for our patients relates to behaviour change. With an ageing population globally, and a clear connection between retaining teeth, quality of life, and general health outcomes, preventative dental care is paramount (Atanda et al., 2021; United Nations Department of Economic and Social Affairs, 2023). Coaching as a means of promoting oral health and fostering behaviour change that supports it has been shown to be effective (Chunda et al., 2023). Further, it aligns well with a philosophy of patient-centred care (Vernon and Howard, 2015). Dentists who learn and apply coaching skills in this way are better equipped to assist their patients in establishing and maintaining sound preventative regimens. Interestingly, some evidence suggests that coaching can also improve the acquisition of these types of skills when delivered alongside more traditional means of healthcare training (Croffoot et al., 2010; Rafferty et al., 2023).

Aside from the primary remit of patient care, dentists also assume the role of team leader in a clinical environment. Indeed, effective leadership has been identified as "critical for success" at all levels of dental practice (Carr et al., 2023). Coaching skills, awareness, and empathy have all been documented as important facets of a leadership in dentistry. Leading with a coaching philosophy also appears to have a ripple effect on our colleagues; they integrate a coaching style into their work which ultimately leads to improvements in team performance (Dong et al., 2022). The role of coaching in developing these leadership competencies in dental residents has also been recognised (Radwan et al., 2023). For dentists who have a role in clinical supervision, coaching may also help to prevent the overbearing micromanagement of students or mentees. This form of clinical supervision has been shown to be unproductive and hinders the learning of our colleagues. Coaching may help foster an approach marked by trust, autonomy, and clear communication (Lee et al., 2023).

In summary, on a professional level, coaching offers opportunities for dentists to progress their clinical skills, deliver more patient-centred care, and be a better leader to their colleagues.

Personal Development

The distinction between personal and professional development is useful for the purposes of explanation but arbitrary in that the two are inextricably linked. Our personal development supports our growth as professionals. Some of the more personal attributes that coaching has been shown to develop include:

- Authenticity
- Resilience
- Processing difficult emotions

Authenticity, albeit a tricky construct to categorically define, implies an awareness of who we are and the self-assuredness to act in accordance with our values, even when external influences challenge them (Jongman-Sereno and Leary, 2019; van den Bosch and Taris, 2014). Coaching invariably involves self-reflection and introspection as a coach guides the conversation with thoughtful questioning. It is not surprising then that coaching research has considered client authenticity as an outcome measure, some documenting advancements in the same (Jackson, 2019; Susing et al., 2011). These findings are significant as cultivating authenticity is related to a plethora of psychological benefits. It has been associated with higher self-esteem, more positive affect, a more hopeful outlook, and protects against depression, anxiety, and stress (Harter, 2002; Luthar et al., 2021; Song et al., 2023; Wood et al., 2008). At work, it has been linked to job satisfaction, in-role performance and work engagement and is negatively associated with workaholism (van den Bosch and Taris, 2014; Vitiello et al., 2016). If we can develop our sense of authenticity, we are likely to experience greater well-being and have a more positive relationship with our work. What's more, authenticity also lies at the heart of patient-centred care by supporting a central component, the patient-doctor relationship. Carl Rogers, one of the forefathers of humanistic psychology and a proponent of person-centred theory, emphasised the importance of what he termed therapist congruence in a patient-therapist relationship (Rogers, 1959). Therapist congruence has been described as genuineness, non-phoniness, and is largely analogous to authenticity (Kolden et al., 2018). As we strengthen our ability to remain authentic in our capacity as professionals, the relationships we build with our patients also become stronger.

Some of the most extensive and highest-quality research into coaching in healthcare settings has investigated resilience (Dyrbye et al., 2023; Fainstad et al., 2022; McGonagle et al., 2020). Given that dentistry has been labelled "one of the most stressful professions" and the high prevalence of burnout in the sector, fostering resilience is perhaps one of the most profound benefits we stand to gain through coaching (Avramova, 2023; Carvalho et al., 2021; Collin et al., 2019; Gorter and Freeman, 2011). Resilience can be defined as an adaptive response to stress, the ability to bounce back and re-establish mental health after exposure to significant adversity (Kunzler et al., 2020; Maunder et al., 2023; Smith et al., 2020). Coaching has been shown to bolster resilience in American surgeons and primary care physicians, with associated reductions in burnout scores (Boet et al., 2023). Resilience is also associated with better overall and mental health in dental students and, in parallel, improved life satisfaction in medical students, higher sleep quality as well as reduced stress, anxiety, and depression in nurses (Lin et al., 2023; Smith et al., 2020; Wang et al., 2022; Wu et al., 2023). While dental-specific evidence is limited, the existing data suggests that resilience promotes our well-being and that coaching has the potential to enhance the resilience of dental practitioners as it has done with our medical colleagues.

Some contemporary research on resilience suggests that the experience of adversity is pivotal in its development (Fox et al., 2018). The emotions that come with adversity can be difficult to process. Learning to navigate them is another facet of personal development that coaching can expedite. Many coaches are familiar with the work of influential psychologists Donald Winnicott and Alfred Bion and their respective theories of "holding" and "containment" (Cox et al., 2023). These concepts refer to the creation of a relationship and environment that is characterised by trust and non-judgement. In these conditions, a coachee is more likely to feel comfortable re-engaging with adverse experiences and challenging emotions. This type of coaching can yield profound insight and facilitate the evolution of adaptive strategies. This personal attribute complements our professional remit as practising dentistry can confront clinicians with a wide range of difficult emotions. As mentioned in the previous section, encountering clinical complications is a reality of dental practice. Further, during our careers, we will encounter patients that we are unable to satisfy. These unpleasant scenarios can precipitate emotions of apathy, frustration, sadness, and guilt in dental practitioners. Refining our ability to recognise and manage these emotions is critical to protecting our well-being and building a career in dentistry that is not only sustainable but engaging and fulfilling.

How Can I Get Started with Coaching?

Before you engage with coaching, perhaps the first point to consider is yourself. Coaching requires a commitment to the process and an openness to honest self-reflection and accountability, which *might* be uncomfortable at times. Literature from the neighbouring field of psychotherapy suggests that client factors like readiness for change is the most important in determining the outcome (McKenna and Davis, 2009). So before you decide to start, make sure it is the right time for you.

Once you have decided to do some coaching, the next step is to find the right coach. One of the issues facing coaching is that it is not a protected title; there is no requirement for coaches to be registered with a regulatory body. "Untrained coaches" have been identified as a significant issue in the field that can undermine its professional legitimacy (Athanasopoulou and Dopson, 2018, p. 70). However, several accreditation bodies exist that have been created to unify coaches globally, establish best practice, and assist clients in finding coaches who share their ethos. The most well-known groups are:

- The International Coaching Federation (ICF)
- The European Mentoring and Coaching Council (EMCC)
- The Association for Coaching (AC)

Each of their websites has a coaching directory that can serve as a useful starting point in finding the right coach for you.

While the activities of these bodies are certainly a step in the right direction, they have occasionally been criticised. Some authors have questioned the empirical validity of "best practice" competency frameworks, highlighting a widening division between academia and the professional bodies and the lack of "cross-fertilisation of ideas" between the two (Bachkirova and Smith, 2015, p. 126). These criticisms have been matched with calls to prioritise university-led qualifications that emphasise objectivity, empiricism, and critical thinking, a stark contrast to the "short-course" format that seems to predominate the coaching sector currently. Accordingly, it is prudent to familiarise yourself with a coach's level of qualification. While there is great diversity in the backgrounds of coaching practitioners, you can expect a formal qualification in coaching itself, ranging from a short-course or postgraduate certificate to master's or doctorate degrees.

While it is the author's view that education is integral to becoming an effective coach, level of experience is also important. In many ways, coaching is a skill-based profession and the integration of academic knowledge into real-time coaching conversations takes practice. Despite the limitations of the accreditation bodies, they typically categorise coaches by hours of practical experience which can be a useful yardstick.

Having reviewed the accreditation, qualification, and experience levels of available coaches, the next step is to schedule a meeting. Many coaches offer an introductory session for prospective clients. The goal of this session is not necessarily to get started and dive into coaching, but rather establish if coaching is the right fit for you; is it likely to successfully address the issues you are facing? These chemistry sessions are also a good opportunity to get a sense of who your coach is. What is their approach? Do they lean more toward one coaching tradition over another? Do you like them? Do you think you could trust them? Have they worked with similar people in the past and is this important to you? In essence, the first meeting is a chance to road test the relationship that you are likely to develop with this person. This is an important step as the coaching relationship is critical in determining the outcome of your sessions (Graßmann et al., 2020). Having met them, you are in a much better position to decide they are the right person to coach you. Following these practical steps will hopefully provide some structure when contemplating coaching.

While emotional intelligence is not the primary focus of this piece, the personal and professional attributes highlighted closely relate to elements of the emotional capital framework discussed elsewhere. Coaching is one avenue to explore in the development of emotional intelligence.

References

Aboalshamat K, Al-Zaidi D, Jawa D, et al. (2020). The effect of life coaching on psychological distress among dental students: Interventional study. *BMC Psychol, 8*(1), 1–106.
Adams J (1988). Coaching: A management style that really gets results. *Dent Manage, 28*(7), 54–57.

Atanda A, Livinski A, Weatherspoon D, Fontelo P, Boroumand S (2021). The impact of tooth retention on health and quality of life in older adults. *Innov Aging*, *5*(Supplement_1), 609–610.

Athanasopoulou A, Dopson S (2018). A systematic review of executive coaching outcomes: Is it the journey or the destination that matters the most? *Leadership Q*, *29*(1), 70–88.

Avramova N (2023). Self-perceived sources of stress and burnout determinants in dentistry – A systematic review. *Galician Med J*, *30*(1), E202317.

Bachkirova T, Smith CL (2015). From competencies to capabilities in the assessment and accreditation of coaches. *Int J Evidence Based Coaching Mentoring*, *13*(2), 123–140.

Boet S, Etherington C, Dion P-M, et al. (2023). Impact of coaching on physician wellness: A systematic review. *PLOS ONE*, *18*(2), e0281406.

Boyatzis RE, Jack AI (2018). The neuroscience of coaching. *Consult Psychol J*, *70*(1), 11–27.

Burt D, Talati Z (2017). The unsolved value of executive coaching: A meta-analysis of outcomes using randomised control trial studies. *Int J Evidence Based Coaching Mentoring*, *15*(2), 17–24.

Carr EO, Park NI, Griggs JA, Koka S (2023). Role of gender and age in influencing dentist perceptions of effective leadership capabilities. *J Prosthetic Dent*, S0022-3913(23)00266-4. doi:10.1016/j.prosdent.2023.04.011.

Carvalho F, Cabaços C, Carneiro M, et al. (2021). Mindfulness and self-compassion based intervention program to prevent burnout in medical and dentistry students. *Eur Psychiatry*, *64*(S1), S459–S460.

Caruso DR, Salovey P (2004). *The Emotionally Intelligent Manager: How to Develop and Use the Four Key Emotional Skills of Leadership*. Jossey-Bass.

Chai HH, Gao SS, Chen KJ, et al. (2021). A concise review on qualitative research in dentistry. *Int J Environmental Res Public Health*, *18*(3), 942.

Chunda R, Mossey P, Freeman R, Yuan S (2023). Health coaching-based interventions for oral health promotion: A scoping review. *Dent J*, *11*(3), 73.

Clear J (2018). *Atomic Habits: An Easy & Proven Way to Build Good Habits & Break Bad Ones*. Penguin/Random House.

Collin V, Toon M, O'Selmo E, Reynolds L, Whitehead P (2019). A survey of stress, burnout and well-being in UK dentists. *Br Dent J*, *226*(1), 40–49.

Cox E, Bachkirova T, Clutterbuck DA (2023). *The Complete Handbook of Coaching*. SAGE Publications.

Croffoot C, Bray K, Black K, Koerber MA (2010). Evaluating the effects of coaching to improve motivational interviewing skills of dental hygiene students. *J Dent Hygiene*, *84*(2), 57–64.

Davidson RJ, McEwen BS (2012). Social influences on neuroplasticity: Stress and interventions to promote well-being. *Nat Neurosci*, *15*(5), 689–695.

Doidge N (2007). *The Brain That Changes Itself: Stories of Personal Triumph from the Frontiers of Brain Science*. Viking.

Dong Y, Dong H, Yuan Y, Jiang J (2022). Role of peer coaching in transmitting the benefits of leader coaching. *Front Psychol*, *12*, 679370.

Dweck CS (2017). *Mindset: Changing The Way You Think to Fulfil Your Potential*. Robinson.

Dyrbye LN, Gill PR, Satele DV, West CP (2023). Professional coaching and surgeon well-being: A randomized controlled trial. *Ann Surg*, *277*(4), 565–571.

Fainstad T, Mann A, Suresh K, et al. (2022). Effect of a novel online group-coaching program to reduce burnout in female resident physicians: A randomized clinical trial. *JAMA Network Open*, *5*(5), e2210752.

Fix GM, VanDeusen Lukas C, Bolton RE, et al. (2018). Patient-centred care is a way of doing things: How healthcare employees conceptualize patient-centred care. *Health Expectations*, *21*(1), 300–307.

Fox S, Lydon S, Byrne D, et al. (2018). A systematic review of interventions to foster physician resilience. *Postgrad Med J*, *94*(1109), 162–170.

Goleman D (1995). *Emotional Intelligence*. Bantam Books.

Gorter RC, Freeman R (2011). Burnout and engagement in relation with job demands and resources among dental staff in Northern Ireland: Burnout and engagement. *Community Dent Oral Epidemiol*, *39*(1), 87–95.

Grant AM, Atad OI (2022). Coaching psychology interventions vs. positive psychology interventions: The measurable benefits of a coaching relationship. *J Positive Psychol*, *7*(4), 532–544.

Graßmann C, Schölmerich F, Schermuly CC (2020). The relationship between working alliance and client outcomes in coaching: A meta-analysis. *Hum Relat*, *73*(1), 35–58.

Harter S (2002). Authenticity. In Snyder CR, Lopez SJ, eds. *Handbook of Positive Psychology*, Oxford University Press; 382–394.

Hauge SM, Willumsen T, Stora B (2022). Dentist-administered CBT for dental anxiety. In Willumsen T, Lein JPA, Gorter RC, Myran L, eds. *Oral Health Psychology: Psychological Aspects Related to Dentistry*, Springer; 195–207.

Hölzel BK, Carmody J, Vangel M, et al. (2011). Mindfulness practice leads to increases in regional brain grey matter density. *Psychiatry Res*, *191*(1), 36–43.

Hwang CY, Kang S-W, Choi SB (2023). Coaching leadership and creative performance: A serial mediation model of psychological empowerment and constructive voice behavior. *Front Psychol*, *14*, 1077594.

International Coaching Federation. (2023). *Global Coaching Study: 2023 Executive Summary*. International Coaching Federation. Accessed Apr 2024 from https://coachingfederation.org/app/uploads/2023/04/2023ICFGlobalCoachingStudy_ExecutiveSummary.pdf?utm_source=ActiveCampaign&utm_medium=email&utm_content=Here+is+Your+Free+Access+to+the+%22ICF+Global+Coaching+Study+2023%22+Executive+Summary&utm_campaign=GCS+Executive+Summary+Delivery&vgo_ee=QJGHP%2BQcYqIbVFLU1NrKpqKesnHFBHCvoUa2Rso615Kdmmn3ykk%3D%3ARoFfY7p5X741KbRBfSEDMgA%2FiPd8vWDr

Jackson S (2019). Coaching women towards authenticity: An appropriate workplace environment. *Int J Evidence Based Coaching Mentoring*, *17*(2), 64–78.

Jongman-Sereno KP, Leary MR (2019). The enigma of being yourself: A critical examination of the concept of authenticity. *Rev Gen Psychol*, *23*(1), 133–142.

Khwaja M (2023). *Resilience and Well-Being for Dental Professionals*. John Wiley & Sons Ltd.

Kolden GG, Wang CC, Austin SB, Chang Y, Klein MH (2018). Congruence/Genuineness: A meta-analysis. *Psychotherapy*, *55*(4), 424–433.

Kunzler AM, Helmreich I, Chmitorz A, et al. (2020). Psychological interventions to foster resilience in healthcare professionals. *Cochrane Database Syst Rev*, *7*(7), CD012527.

Lee J, Ahn S, Henning MA, van de Ridder JMM, Rajput V (2023). Micromanagement in clinical supervision: A scoping review. *BMC Med Educ*, *23*(1), 563–563.

Lin YE, Lin CT, Hu ML, Tzeng S, Chien LY (2023). The relationships among perceived stress, resilience, sleep quality and first-month retention of newly employed nurses: A cross-sectional survey. *Nursing Open*, *10*(6), 4004–4012.

Luthar SS, Ebbert AM, Kumar NL (2021). Risk and resilience among Asian American youth: Ramifications of discrimination and low authenticity in self-presentations. *Am Psychol*, *76*(4), 643–657.

Maragha T, Donnelly L, Schuetz C, Bergmann H, Brondani M (2023). Students' resilience and mental health in the dental curriculum. *Eur J Dent Educ*, *27*(1), 174–180.

Maunder RG, Rosen B, Heeney ND, et al. (2023). Relationship between three aspects of resilience-adaptive characteristics, withstanding stress, and bouncing back-in hospital workers exposed to prolonged occupational stress during the COVID-19 pandemic: A longitudinal study. *BMC Health Serv Res*, *23*(1), 703.

McGonagle AK, Schwab L, Yahanda N, et al. (2020). Coaching for primary care physician well-being: A randomized trial and follow-up analysis. *J Occup Health Psychol*, *25*(5), 297–314.

McKenna DD, Davis SL (2009). Hidden in plain sight: The active ingredients of executive coaching. *Ind Organ Psychol*, *2*(3), 244–260.

Mead N, Bower P (2000). Patient-centredness: A conceptual framework and review of the empirical literature. *Soc Sci Med*, *51*(7), 1087–1110.

Merzenich M (2013). *Soft-Wired: How the New Science of Brain Plasticity Can Change Your Life*. Parnassus Publishing.

Metzger Samuels CT (1991). Mentoring: An administrative perspective. *J Dent Educ*, *55*(10), 671–672.

Murariu A, Balcoş C, Bobu L, et al. (2019). Coaching in dentistry – A literature review. *Romanian J Med Dent Educ*, *8*(11), 55–61.

Neff K (2003). Self-compassion: An alternative conceptualization of a healthy attitude toward oneself. *Self Identity*, *2*(2), 85–101.

Pinkham JR (1993). Ontological coaching and the "rules of the game". *J California Dent Assoc*, *21*(4), 48.

Plessas A, Paisi M, Bryce M, et al. (2022). Mental health and well-being interventions in the dental sector: A systematic review. *Evidence-Based Dent*, 1–8. doi:10.1038/s41432-022-0831-0.

Radwan H, Al-Nasser S, Alzahem A (2023). Developing leadership among dental residents: An exploratory study. *Curēus*, *15*(3), e36600.

Rafferty R, Fairbrother G, Cashin A (2023). Maximising leadership coaching training outcomes: A randomised controlled trial. *Int J Evidence Based Coaching Mentoring*, *21*(2), 146–161.

Rogers CR (1959). A Theory of Therapy, Personality, and Interpersonal Relationships: As Developed in the Client-Centered Framework. In Koch S, ed., *Psychology: A Study of a Science*. McGraw-Hill; 3, 184–256.

Schneider S, Kingsolver K, Rosdahl J (2014). Physician coaching to enhance well-being: A qualitative analysis of a pilot intervention. *Explore*, *10*(6), 372–379.

Smith CS, Carrico CK, Goolsby S, Hampton AC (2020). An analysis of resilience in dental students using the resilience scale for adults. *J Dent Educ*, *84*(5), 566–577.

Song L, Zheng J, Li F, et al. (2023). Neurostructural correlates of trait authenticity: Increased surface area in the left precuneus and decreased volume in the left amygdala. *Pers Individ Differ*, *208*, 112193.

Stormon N, Sexton C, Ford PJ, Eley DS (2022). Understanding the well-being of dentistry students. *Eur J Dent Educ*, *26*(1), 1–10.

Susing I, Green LS, Grant AM (2011). The potential use of the authenticity scale as an outcome measure in executive coaching. *Coaching Psychol*, *7*(1), 16–25.

Theeboom T, Beersma B, van Vianen AEM (2014). Does coaching work? A meta-analysis on the effects of coaching on individual level outcomes in an organizational context. *J Positive Psychol*, *9*(1), 1–18.

United Nations Department of Economic and Social Affairs (2023). *World Social Report 2023: Leaving No One Behind in an Ageing World*. Accessed Apr 2024 from https://www.un.org/development/desa/dspd/wp-content/uploads/sites/22/2023/01/WSR_2023_Chapter_Key_Messages.pdf

van den Bosch R, Taris TW (2014). Authenticity at work: Development and validation of an individual authenticity measure at work. *J Happiness Stud*, *15*(1), 1–18.

van Niewerburgh C (2012). *Coaching in Education: Getting Better Results for Students, Educators, and Parents*. Routledge.

Vernon LT, Howard AR (2015). Advancing health promotion in dentistry: Articulating an integrative approach to coaching Oral health behavior change in the dental setting. *Curr Oral Health Rep*, *2*(3), 111–122.

Vitiello K, Aziz S, Wuensch KL (2016). Workaholism and authenticity: The role of life satisfaction. *J Behav Appl Manage*, *17*(2), 116.

Wang Q, Sun W, Wu H (2022). Associations between academic burnout, resilience and life satisfaction among medical students: A three-wave longitudinal study. *BMC Med Educ*, *22*(1), 248–248.

Whitmore J (2009). *Coaching for Performance: Growing Human Potential and Purpose: the Principles and Practice of Coaching and Leadership*, 4th ed. Nicholas Brealey.

Willumsen T, Lein JPA, Gorter RC, Myran L (2022). *Oral Health Psychology: Psychological Aspects Related to Dentistry*. Springer.

Wood AM, Linley PA, Maltby J, Baliousis M, Joseph S (2008). The authentic personality: A theoretical and empirical conceptualization and the development of the authenticity scale. *J Couns Psychol*, *55*(3), 385–399.

Wu CF, Liu TH, Cheng CH, Chang KY (2023). Relationship between nurses' resilience and depression, anxiety and stress during the 2021 COVID-19 outbreak in Taiwan. *Nurs Open*, *10*(3), 1592–1600.

Index

Note: **Bold** page numbers refer to **tables** and in *italics* to figures.

ethical standards, 43
measured responses to stress, 42
positive workplace relationships, 43
Hülsheger, U.R., 34

I

Impulsive reactions, 29
Ineffective conflict management, 79–80
Interpersonal relationships, 29–30

K

Kelm, Z., 66

L

Leadership, 69, 83, 113
Levinson, W., 62
Litigation, 61–62
Lower team cohesion, 60
Low self-control, 43
  compromised ethics, 43
  difficult interpersonal relationships, 43
  difficulty handling stress, 43
  impulsiveness, 43
  poor time management, 43

M

Maslow, A.H., 89–90, 92, 96
Mayer, J.D., 2, 11
McEwen, B.S., 103
Meditation, 45–46
Mentorship, 82
Merzenich, M., 104
Mindfulness, 45–46, 64
Miscommunication, 59
Multi-source feedback (MSF), 18
Myers, H.L., 8
Myers, L.B., 8

N

National Health Service (NHS) dental
  practices, 1, 4, 5, 16
Neff, K.D., 63
Neuroplasticity, 103

New behaviours, 103–104
  rewiring your brain, 103–104
Newman, Dr Martyn, 28, 30
Non-verbal communication, 108

O

Open communication, 50, 68
Optimism, 4
Optimistic future, 5

P

Patient-centred care, 74, 83, 112
Patient-centred communication, 67
Patient expectations, 7
Patient satisfaction, 59
Peer support, 82
  groups, 64
Personal goals, 46
Personal insight, 29
Physical activity, 46
Plato, 57, 77
Poor communication, 79
Positive change, 103
  success factors, 103, 105–106
Positive work environment, 59
Practical recommendations, 103
Practice active listening, 108
Practice management, costs, 8
Practitioner perspective, 103
Professional counselling or therapy, 65
Professional development, 69
Professional practice, 2
Psychological safety, 4, 33

R

Realistic expectations, 64–65
Recognition, 83
Reflective learning, 29
Reflective practice, 68
Regulatory and legal pressures, 8
Relationship skills, 4, *23*, 77–84
  definition of, 78–80
  dental practitioner perspective, 85–88
  dental students, 80
  developing, 82–84